NINETEENTH CENTURY
AMERICAN COLOR PLATE BOOKS

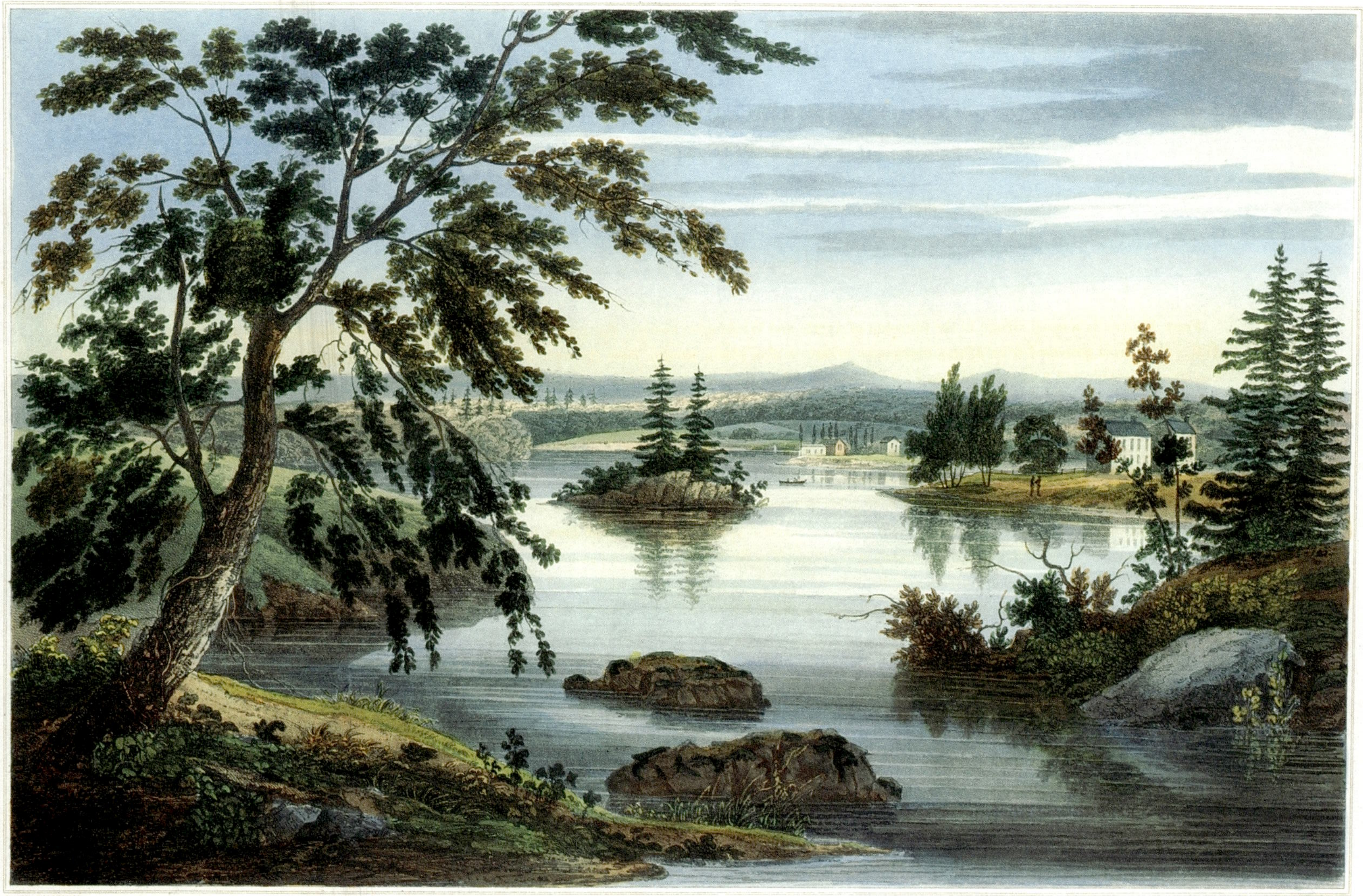

PAINTED BY W. G. WALL. ENGRAVED BY J. HILL.

VIEW NEAR FORT MILLER.

No. 10 of the Hudson River Port Folio

Published by Henry I. Megarey New York

Stamped with a National Character:

NINETEENTH CENTURY AMERICAN COLOR PLATE BOOKS

AN EXHIBITION

WILLIAM S. REESE

NEW YORK: THE GROLIER CLUB 1999

This catalogue was published to accompany an exhibition
at The Grolier Club, May 4–July 31, 1999.

ISBN 0-910-627-27-X

Illustrated on front cover:
Item 84, [Walker], *Statistical Atlas of the United States*... (chromolithograph).

Illustrated opposite:
Item 2, Birch, *The Country Seats of the United States*... (hand-colored copper plate engraving).

Illustrated on back cover:
Item 6, Wall, *The Hudson River Portfolio* (aquatint with hand coloring).

Photography by Joseph Szaszfai.

Printed in Italy. Designed and produced in New York by Ink, Inc.

TO MY MOTHER AND FATHER

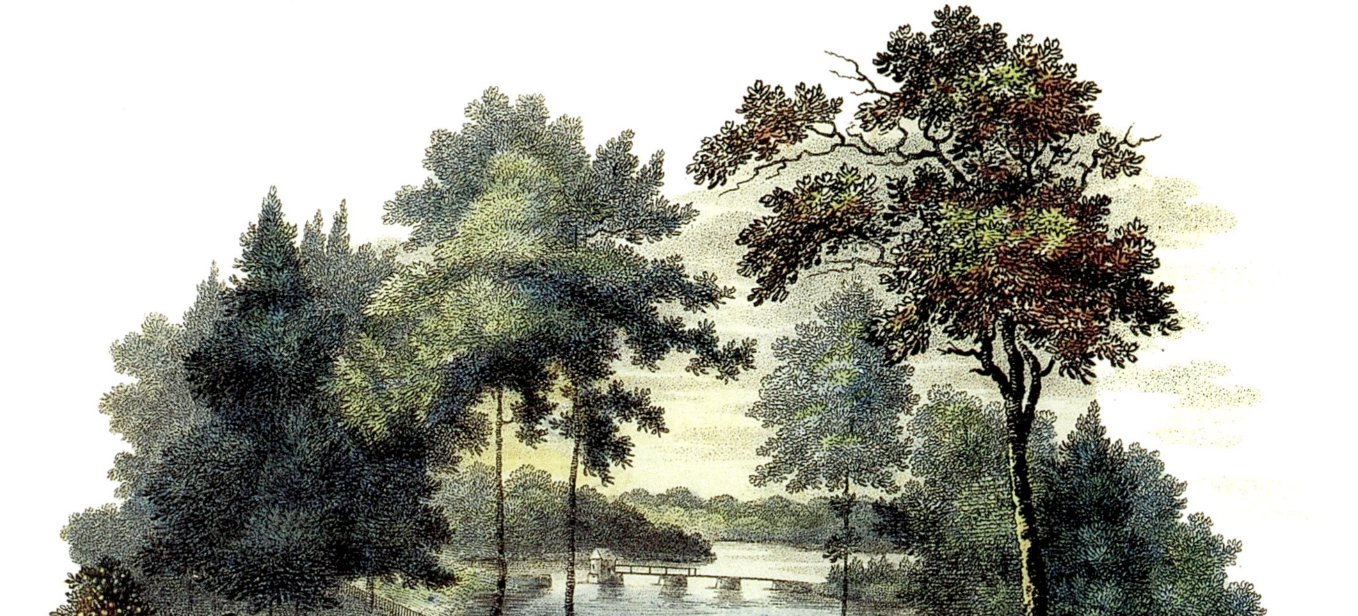

CONTENTS

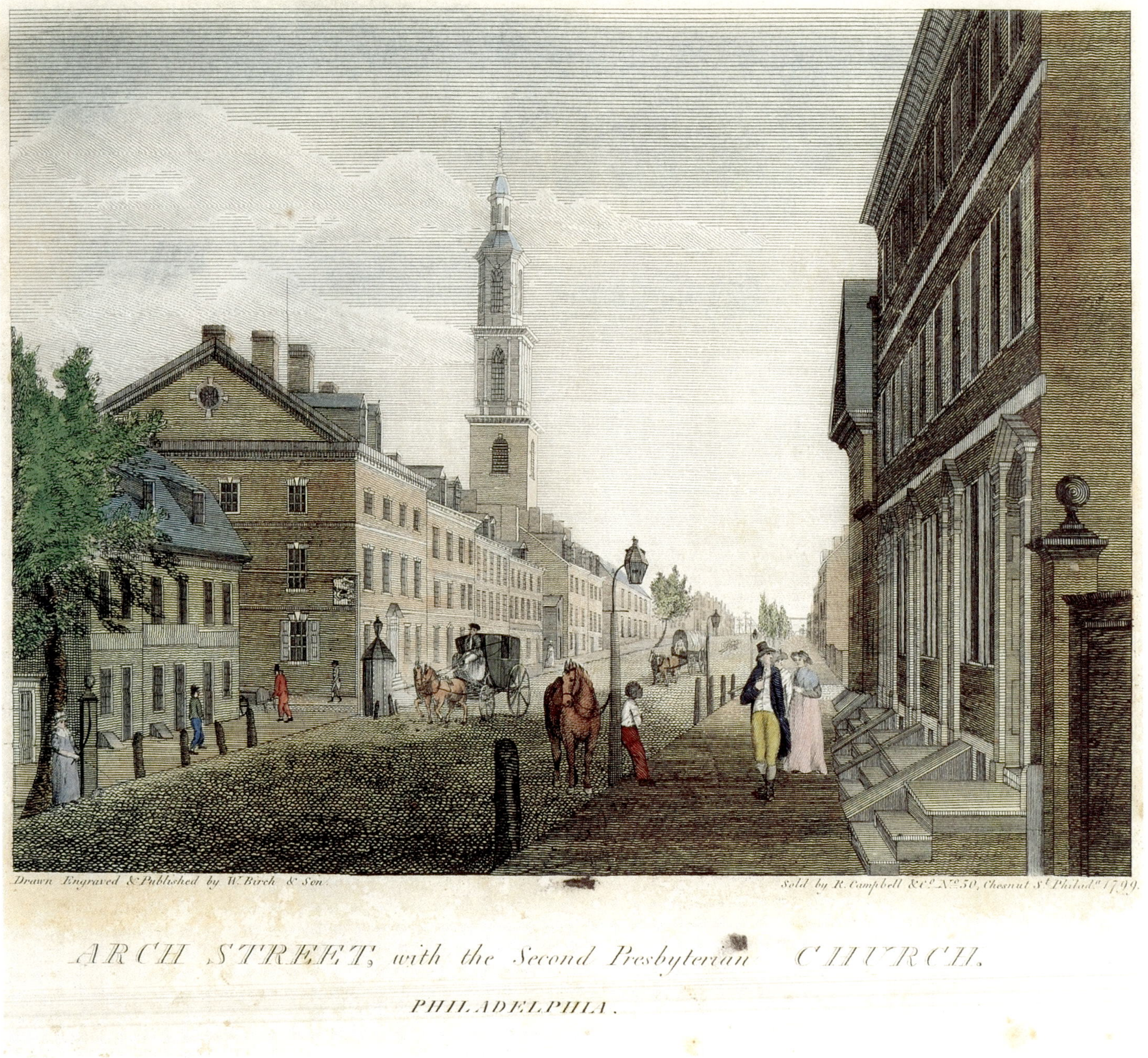

1. Birch, *The City of Philadelphia....*
Hand-colored copper plate engraving.

THIS EXHIBITION traces the history and development of American color plate books in the 19th century. Historical events seldom create neat time periods, but in this case the century fairly defines an era. The first American color plate book, William Birch's *The City of Philadelphia... As It Appeared in the Year 1800*, was published in parts in 1799–1800. At the end of the century, the mid-1890s saw the dawn of the widespread use of the trichromatic half-tone process, which quickly replaced the various mediums for producing color plate book illustrations that had been in use throughout the preceding century. This technological revolution introduced the methods which would dominate color illustration for most of the 20th century and provides a terminal point for this exhibition. From Birch to the color halftone, color plate books evolved from being produced almost exclusively by hand to being almost entirely manufactured by machine. The chief means of production passed from hand-colored copper plate engravings, aquatints, and lithographs, to the introduction and development of chromolithography. Experiments with some more exotic processes were also undertaken before the rise of photomechanical printing made them all obsolete. The 19th century encompasses the birth, rise, and ultimate demise of these methods of production in the culture of printed books in America.

At the end of the 20th century, we are so accustomed to seeing color in every publication that it seems commonplace. The color revolution of the digital age has moved so rapidly that it is easy to forget how expensive, and consequently how sparingly, it was used in book illustration just a generation ago. To understand the books in this exhibition, the viewer must remember that in the 19th century color in books represented luxury. Although advances in technology made color plates steadily more accessible to a wider (and increasingly affluent) audience, there was never a time when color was cheap. The big color plate books were extremely costly and only available to the rich. The modest uses of color in gift books and the like were a small taste of the lavish life for the less affluent. Book buyers wanted color and publishers strove to supply it. New methods steadily made color more affordable, primarily by substituting mechanical work for hand finishing, often at the cost of quality. The balance between the cost of production and the potential market largely determined what was published.

This exhibition explores a world of lost processes and skills. There are no printers with the ability to produce such works in aquatint or chromolithography today, although many of the media are still used by contemporary artists. The show traces the progression of these processes and the careers of some of the leading practitioners. It also attempts to view the uses 19th-century Americans chose to make of color illustration in books in a broad variety of fields, both to instruct and amuse.

Two major genres of color illustration in books are deliberately excluded from this exhibition: children's books and cartography. This was not done because of a lack of understanding of their importance. Both are major fields of color book illustration, and both encompass enough material for fascinating exhibitions on their own. The two fields have long-standing separate traditions of collecting, bibliography, and scholarship, and it seemed best, given the space limitations, to leave their story to be told in full by someone totally conversant with the topics so they may be done the justice they deserve. Since these fields were already distinct in the 19th century and generally involved specialist publishers, I do not think their exclusion here harms the narration of the larger story of 19th-century American color plate books.

What is an American Color Plate Book?

At first glance, the definition of a 19th-century American color plate book seems quite simple, but in fact the term is fraught with ambiguity. Only the chronological element is indisputable. In my interpretation, the first requirement of "American" is that the plates themselves were printed and colored in the Americas. This theoretically includes the entire Western Hemisphere, but in practice almost always means the United States. Color plate books were produced on a limited scale in Canada beginning in 1838. Some extraordinary books were produced in Latin America and the Caribbean, most notably in Havana, Mexico City, Rio de Janeiro, and Lima (for examples, see items 85 through 88 in the catalogue). However, the overwhelming percentage of imprints are from the United States, so that "American" can be taken as virtually synonymous with being printed in the United States.

Books with color plates printed and colored in Europe are not American color plate books. This obviously excludes books *about* America published in Europe, such as Karl Bodmer's famous atlas illustrating the travels of Prince Maximilian of Wied. It is more difficult to detect works with American imprints, often with letterpress text printed in America, that use imported plates. These include such notable books as A. J. Downing's *The Fruits and Fruit Trees of America* (New York, 1850), whose hand-colored engravings were produced in Paris; Edward Beyer's *Album of Virginia* (Richmond, 1858), whose tinted lithographs were printed in Dusseldorf; George W. Kendall's *The War Between the United States and Mexico Illustrated* (New York, 1851), whose hand-colored lithographs were imported from Paris while the letterpress was printed in New Orleans; and Capt. F. Brinkley's *Japan, Described and Illustrated by the Japanese* (Boston, 1897), whose hand-colored photographic plates were actually manufactured in Tokyo. These are only some of the more prominent examples, easily detectable because the place of printing is clearly stated on the plate or in the text. Others give themselves away by their style: for example, the books published by the Philadelphia firm of Weik have plates which appear clearly to be from Germany, although this is never stated and all of their books have a Philadelphia imprint.

The frequency of these false imprints demonstrates an aspect of the most important theme in the history of the American color plate book: the influence of European color printing on American work. European plates were imported either because they were better or cheaper than American work, or sometimes both. They were also used because the medium the author or the publisher desired was simply not available in the United States. Thus Daniel G. Elliot was driven to commission the plates for his later works in London and Brussels because Bowen & Co., who produced those of his first three books, went out of business in 1870, leaving no other American printer capable of making hand-colored lithographs of the quality Elliot demanded and on the scale he envisioned.

European work also crossed the Atlantic in the form of printing plates, and these are considered American color plates, since they were printed and colored in the United States. The most notable examples of these are the Redouté plates for Michaux's *North American Sylva* (item 21), cut and first printed in Paris, but later imported and used for editions in Cincinnati and Philadelphia.

The question of what constitutes color in a plate is also open to interpretation. In the era of copper plates and aquatint, this is seldom a question: plates were usually colored by hand or not at all. The advent of the tinted lithograph and the beginnings of chromolithography in the early 1840s complicates the issue. How many tints make the plate a "color" plate? Generally, three tints besides the original printing of the image, or several tints with added hand coloring, are required to consider that a plate is colored. But exceptions prove the rule, and there are cases in which the printer skillfully juxtaposed two tints so as to suggest a greater effect of color.

Earlier bibliographers such as Whitman Bennett and Daniel McGrath arbitrarily set four color plates as the number needed to qualify a work as a color plate book. This is a reasonable standard, since there are a tremendous number of books with a beautifully colored frontispiece, or a few additional color plates, but which are predominantly illustrated in black and white. The color in these books is secondary to their overall makeup. I have adhered to this definition, thus excluding a host of books with only one or two color plates.

Periodicals, strictly speaking, do not qualify as color plate books. The line between books and serials is often blurred by the manner in which a number of works were published. Such publications as *The Cabinet of Natural History* or the Landreths' *The Floral Magazine* were issued in dated monthly issues, with no indication that the publishers did not intend to continue indefinitely. Nonetheless, today they are considered books. The fashion magazines, such as *Frank Leslie's Ladies Gazette* are unquestionably periodicals. I have included them in this exhibition because virtually all American fashion plates appeared in periodicals, and few elsewhere. This was an important aspect of color plate illustration, and such periodicals were frequently preserved and marketed in bound annual volumes.

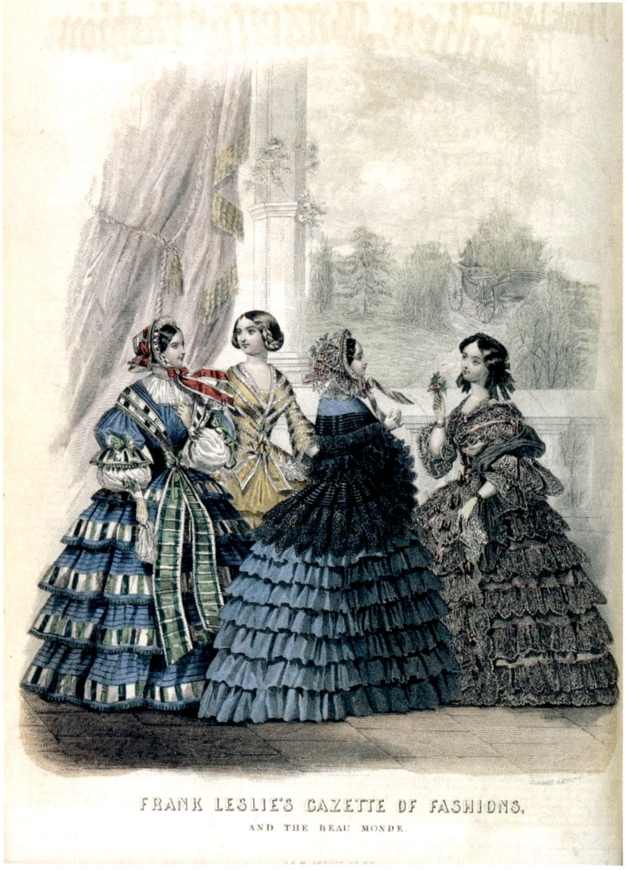

49. Leslie, *Ladies Gazette of Fashion....* Hand-colored steel engraving.

Finally, there is the question of what constitutes a book, a debate certainly far beyond the scope of this exhibition. With material of this sort, the line between a book and a collection of plates is often a thin one. For example, does an accordion-fold panel with twenty-four scenes, all hand-colored, presenting a comic narrative story, issued in a cloth binding, qualify? I do not think it does, but some may disagree. Nor does a series of colored prints, issued and numbered as a sequence, with a narrative text in the caption of each print, but no other unifying text. On the other hand, if that series of prints was ever issued in a bound format with a title page, it does qualify. Ideally, a color plate book is a combination of color illustration and words, with the plates designed to serve as a parallel visual text to interact with and explicate the written text. This function is clear in the vast majority of books in this exhibition. Some genres, such as trade catalogues, have traditionally not been admitted to be books, although in some cases their physical makeup is that of a bound book with title page and plates. I do feel that some of these reasonably qualify, and several have been included in the exhibition (see items 68, 70, 72, 98).

For all of these reasons, it is impossible to fence in the field of 19th-century American color plate books, and quantitative analysis must remain vague as a result. Anyone attempting a definitive bibliography of the field will be plagued by these questions of qualification. Despite this, the major books and important genres seem clear enough, and they are the subject of this show.

The vagaries of defining exactly what constitutes a color plate book increases the difficulty of determining how many were produced in 19th century America. We can, however, venture a reasonable guess. Whitman Bennett, in his pioneering *A Practical Guide to American Nineteenth Century Color Plate Books* (1949), lists 390 works. Although grievously incomplete, this is still the primary bibliographical study of the subject. Bennett includes a number of books with imported plates, but omits such topics as medicine and architecture, as well as the subjects of cartography and children's books which, as noted above, are also excluded from this exhibition. At the time of writing, having intensively collected the genre for the last five years, I have accumulated almost exactly half of the titles listed in Bennett. However, I have about six hundred titles, or fifty percent more than he lists. If we take this ratio as a guide, however rough, it suggests that the universe of 19th-century American color plate books, as defined here and excluding cartography and children's books, contains about 1,200 to 1,500 titles.

The great majority of works qualifying as color plate books are relatively small or have relatively few color plates. Many of the gift book genre, which probably accounts for several hundred of the titles, have only a handful of small plates each. More ambitious projects, such as the large architectural works published in mid-century, are lavishly illustrated, but mainly with tinted plates, having just enough color to qualify. In many other works, color is an enhancement, but not the main thrust of the book. It is fair to say, all told, that not more than ten percent of the universe we have established are large-scale, "serious" color plate books. In other words, the heart and core of 19th-century American color plate books can be found in about 150 titles, about half of which appear in this show.

Relatively few large color plate books were published in 19th century America. Color plate illustrations were expensive and difficult to produce. For much of the century, America lagged behind Europe and constantly looked across the Atlantic for artisans and technology. Ambitious projects frequently foundered for lack of customers. The present rarity of many of the books that were completed suggests they were done in small editions. Other formats of color work were more suited to American tastes and markets.

Despite all this, some extraordinary color plate books were produced in America, all the more remarkable because of the adverse conditions under which they were produced. Ultimately, printers and publishers brought out at least some works that could stand on the same level as the European models they sought to emulate.

Color Printers and Color Plate Books

The story of color printing in 19th-century America is closely linked to that of color plate books, but the two are by no means the same. Some of the leading printers figure in both stories, most notably Peter S. Duval in Philadelphia before the Civil War, and Louis Prang in Boston in the last three decades of the century. Both of these men were innovators who were quick to adopt new technology, as well as entrepreneurs who ran two of the largest printing firms of their eras. Providing color plates for books was a major part of Duval's overall business. For Prang it was less so, since the majority of his large and varied output of art reproductions and ephemeral material was not intended for book illustration. Both were color printers, but Duval was far more concerned with the needs of authors and publishers to illustrate their text than was Prang.

Virtually all of the printers of color plates for book illustration also produced other color work. For most of them, the production of prints, advertising material, trade cards, and the like, was a more important factor in their businesses than were plates for books. At the same time, there were numerous color printers who had little or no involvement with book illustration. Currier & Ives are the most famous of these. The vast majority of colored illustrative material produced in the United States during the 19th century was intended for something other than book illustration, such as individual prints and advertising ephemera. Color plate books were only one aspect of the work of printers producing color work, and it was a specialized subset of the color printing work going on in America. Plates for book illustration do not encompass the full range of American color printing. Rather, they reflect the demands imposed by the texts they illustrate.

The appetite of American audiences was clearly different than that of Europeans in the kinds of color work that were marketable. For example, colored city and country views were very popular in the United States. Thousands were produced, and they were a mainstay of some of the leading lithographers. Yet the American market signally failed to produce the kinds of view books which were so popular in England and Europe. The catalogues by Major John R. Abbey, *Life in England, Scenery of Great Britain and Ireland* and *Travel in Aquatint and Lithography*, give some idea of the number of these European works, which found a sufficient base of financial support from wealthy individuals to finance hundreds of volumes. The few similar projects attempted in America almost invariably failed to attain completion. The two most notable, *Picturesque Views of American Scenery* (item 5) and the *Hudson River Portfolio* (item 6), both ceased publication before all of their projected parts had been issued. Later notable attempts, such as John W. Audubon's *Illustrated Notes of an Expedition Through Mexico and California* (item 41) and George Harvey's *Harvey's Scenes of the Primitive Forests of America,* were originally the pilot numbers for much larger schemes (both were intended to be ten numbers of four plates each) which failed to attract enough subscribers to carry the project beyond the initial number.

Clearly, Americans liked views, but they wanted to buy them to frame and put on the wall, an inexpensive and democratic form of art. The expense of the big view books required a secure, wealthy leisure class with the money to buy them, a library to put them in, and the time to look at them. In England, the aristocracy and moneyed gentry supported such publications. In America, they died aborning, or succeeded to the extent they did because they could also be marketed as individual prints. As evidence of this, it is notable that complete sets of the *Hudson River Portfolio* are extremely rare, although some of the individual prints are fairly common.

The engravers, lithographers, and chromolithographers who produced the color plates generally did so as job work. They seldom acted as the publisher, although there were notable exceptions to this, such as James Ackerman's pirated edition of *Catlin's North American Indian Portfolio* (item 25) and many of Louis Prang's books. P. S. Duval, for example, did not act as publisher of any of the many works in which his plates appeared, although he did publish many individual prints. Authors, artists, or publishers would typically work very closely with the printers they hired. On occasion, such as in the relationship between the Audubon family and James T. Bowen, the customers virtually took over the lithographers with their demands.

Since the publication of most American color plate books was in the hands of authors, publishers, or government agencies, it was their goals, tastes, and pocketbooks which shaped the formats of the books and plates they produced. The boldest productions, such as those of the Audubons, were frequently the result of the author or artist also acting as entrepreneur, taking a financial risk to produce the book they envisioned. The distressing frequency with which these projects failed certainly served to warn printers away from attempting any similar enterprises on their own.

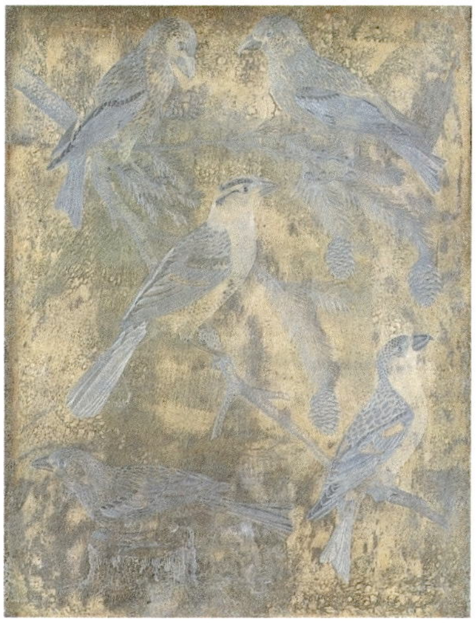

4. Wilson, *American Ornithology....* Original copper plate.

The impact of European craftsmanship and technological innovation on American work cannot be too strongly emphasized. In the first half of the 19th century, the vast majority of artisans working in the field were immigrants. William Birch had moved to Pennsylvania from England in 1794. John Hill, the only real master of aquatint in the United States, had just arrived from England when he undertook his great landscape view books in the 1820s. The engraver, Alexander Lawson, who produced the plates for Alexander Wilson's *American Ornithology*, was trained in Scotland, and even an American-born artist such as Cornelius Tiebout served an apprenticeship in London. Duval had immigrated from France in 1831, and his lithographic business steadily recruited new workmen from France, bringing with them the latest European techniques. William Sharp, the father of chromolithography in the United States, brought the art with him when he moved to Boston in 1841, as is demonstrated by the collection of chromo proofs struck in his native England before his immigration, now in the Boston Public Library.

The revolutions of 1848 drove many skilled Continental craftsmen with liberal political views to immigrate, and brought to America two of the leading figures in chromolithography: Julius Bien to New York and Louis Prang to Boston. In the post-Civil War era, the printing industries in the United States had developed sufficiently that the dependence on European master craftsmen lessened, although the Americans continued to look to French, German, and

British printers for technical advances. For almost the entire century, European craftsmen and technology were a major factor in American color plate work. It was only in the 1870s that the American printers began to forge ahead on their own. The works of Prang and such books as Earhart's *The Color Printer* (item 111) show that, by the end of the century, American printers were finally creating new techniques independent of Europe.

Despite the strong European influence and involvement in the production of American color plates, a number of the major books made strongly nationalistic assertions as part of their justification for publication. William Birch set the tone in the preface to *The City of Philadelphia . . . In the Year 1800*, stating that his goal was to demonstrate to Europe the quality of life in that city, and thereby encourage trade and commerce. John Hill wrote that he wished to display the landscape of America because "Our country abounds with Scenery, comprehending all the varieties of the sublime, the beautiful, and the picturesque in nature. . . ." Fielding Lucas, in the preface to his *Drawing Book,* notes that the book was based on English models, but that he chose American themes for the illustrations "to stamp it with a national character." Many of the early monuments of natural history, such as Wilson's *American Ornithology*, Bigelow's *American Medical Botany*, or Barton's *A Flora of North America*, emphasize American themes. The many books dealing with Native Americans also played upon their national character, even as the subjects were being exterminated.

This sense of national pride as a selling point and justification was brought to its highest point by the Audubons. The octavo *Birds of America* was styled as "The Great National Work," and the later *Quadrupeds* projects were advertised in a similar way. Patriotism seems to have worked as a marketing tool, since the works of Audubon, Michaux and Nuttall, and McKenney and Hall went through multiple editions up to the 1880s.

In the mid-1840s the advent of government sponsored projects added a new element to the themes of nationalism. The Wilkes Expedition, with its numerous atlases of color plates, self-consciously sought to compete with similar projects underwritten by the French and British governments. The Pacific Railroad Surveys furthered the role of government in color plate books, spending huge sums of money on the printing and production of reports. Even private spin-offs, such as Hayden and Moran's *The Yellowstone National Park* (item 99), used a government funded expedition and chauvinistic pride in the wonders of the first national park as the basis for successfully marketing a color plate book.

The twin themes of European craftsmanship in execution and nationalistic pride in the United States as a marketing tool are a peculiar combination. But as the 19th century advanced, the ability of Americans to learn and copy new technology from Europe while exploiting it on wholly American themes produced some beautiful and remarkable books. This interweaving of the crafts of the Old World evolving in the New is at the heart of the story of American color plate books.

Types of Color Plates

As this exhibition includes examples of a number of different technologies of color printing, a brief overview of the prevalent mediums and the time periods in which they were used, may be helpful:

The earliest American color plate books, beginning with the works of William Birch, were illustrated with hand-colored copper plate engravings. This was the preferred medium of most printers before 1830, when lithography rapidly replaced it. It survived for a time in the hands of such veteran artisans as Alexander Lawson, although most other engravers turned to steel plates for their work. However, existing copper plates were often preserved and printed throughout the remaining decades of the century.

Between 1818 and 1827, there was a brief flowering of books illustrated with hand-colored aquatint engraving. This was largely due to the energy of a single man, John Hill, who was responsible for the execution of most of the major aquatint projects. A difficult and expensive process, aquatint never gained widespread use in America, except for the publication of individual prints. Although several stunning books were produced, it was overwhelmed by the advent of lithography, a more cost effective means of book illustration.

In the early period several books experimented with mediums which saw little or no further use in book illustration. Bigelow's *American Medical Botany* (item 10), for example, employed the unusual process of etching on stone, inking the stone with multiple colors applied by hand *a la poupée*, and then printing with a single impression. This laborious process of etching on stone was never used again in an American book, although some were printed using metal plates inked in a similar fashion. Several books, notably Barton's *A Flora of North America* (item 11), employed engravings printed in color and finished by hand. This technique, borrowed (as was Bigelow's stone etching) from continental engravers, never achieved widespread use in America.

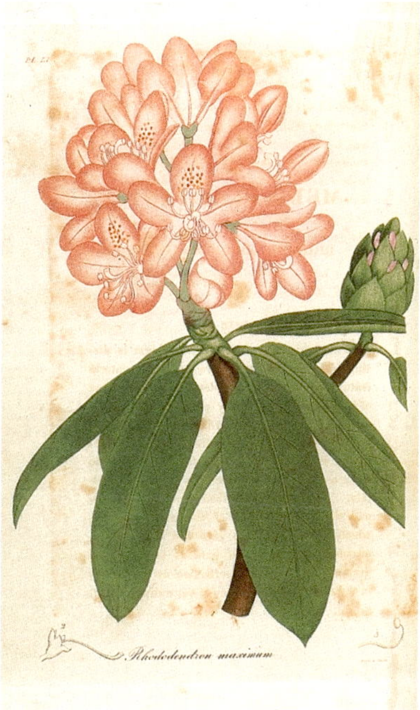

10. Bigelow, *American Medical Botany....* Hand-colored *a la poupée* from etched stone.

Lithography, in various forms, was the dominant medium used in American 19th-century color plate books. First used for book illustration in the United States in 1819, it was employed in ever more complex ways through the end of the century. The vast majority of books in this show have plates produced by some form of the lithographic process.

A few modest books with hand-colored lithographic plates, such as Peter Guillet's *Timber Merchant's Guide*, appeared in the early 1820s. It was not until 1830, when John and Thomas Doughty's *The Cabinet of Natural History* (item 12) began serial publication, that hand-colored lithographs emerged as a primary medium of book illustration. The next two decades were the heyday of the hand-colored lithograph. From 1850 on, the labor and expense involved in producing entirely hand-colored plates slowly lost ground to the developing processes of chromolithography. The last major works using the technique were Daniel G. Elliot's three large folio ornithological works, culminating in

20. Hovey,
The Fruits of America....
Chromolithograph.

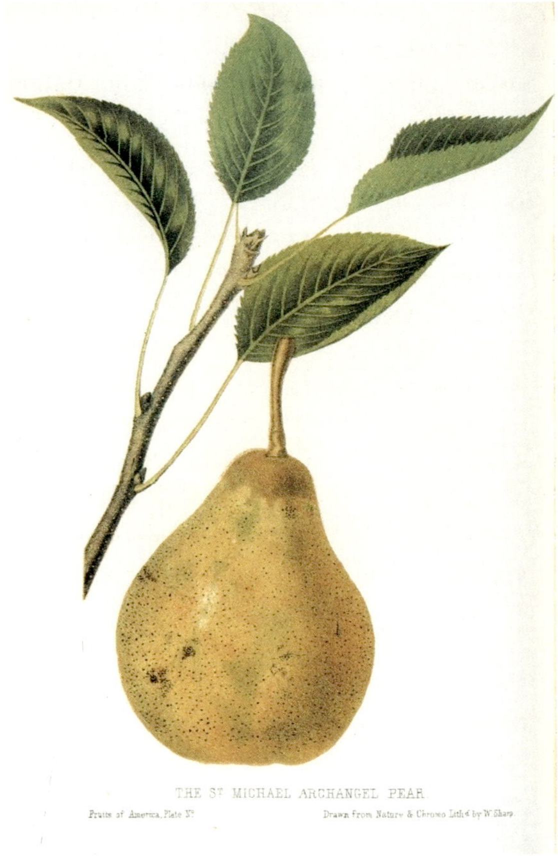

1866–1869 with *The New and Heretofore Unfigured Species of the Birds of North America* (item 44). After the demise of their printer, Bowen & Co., in 1870, only a few scattered works appeared with fully hand-colored plates.

An early labor-saving step in coloring lithographed plates was the use of printed tints. These were employed as early as 1842 by Duval, and soon became common. Many plates in the 1850s and 1860s either featured multiple tints or applied hand coloring on top of one or more tints. Such processes were less expensive than full hand coloring, and developed in tandem with more elaborate chromolithography.

The first American book illustrated with chromolithography was Mattson's *American Vegetable Practice* (item 17), published in 1841. This primitive effort used as many as five different stones and colors to produce color plates that were entirely printed. The problems of registration and inking required considerable expertise to manage, but by 1850 chromolithography was capable of providing mechanically produced book illustrations that rivaled hand-applied color. Hovey's *The Fruits of America* (item 20) was the first major work executed entirely in chromolithography. By the early 1850s, some plates employed as many as ten separate stones to achieve complex color effects. Other printers in this period used hand-finishing in conjunction with chromolithographic plates, most boldly in the Bien edition of Audubon's *Birds* (item 40). By the late 1860s, chromolithography had practically driven out hand coloring as an economically viable medium in book illustration.

In the meantime, hand-colored steel engravings succeeded copper engravings in the 1830s. Most steel engraved plates were intended to be black and white and so do not enter this story. However, hand-colored steel engravings were popular, mainly for fashion plates, in the 1840s and 1850s. Illustrators of fashion also toyed with other esoteric media, including a brief revival of an aquatint process in *The Artist* (item 48) in 1842.

Illustrations printed from wood were also mainly intended to appear in black and white, but there were exceptions. From the 1830s to the 1870s a number of cheap, sloppily colored plates were used in a variety of popular histories and subscription books, such as Trumbull's *History of the Discovery of America* (item 27). These inexpensively produced works were of the poorest order of workmanship. More sophisticated printers experimented with printing color from multiple wood blocks, as in *The Winter Bloom* (item 56) and *The Gallery of Scriptural Engravings* (item 90), with interesting effect. Neither of these more subtle mediums were widely used.

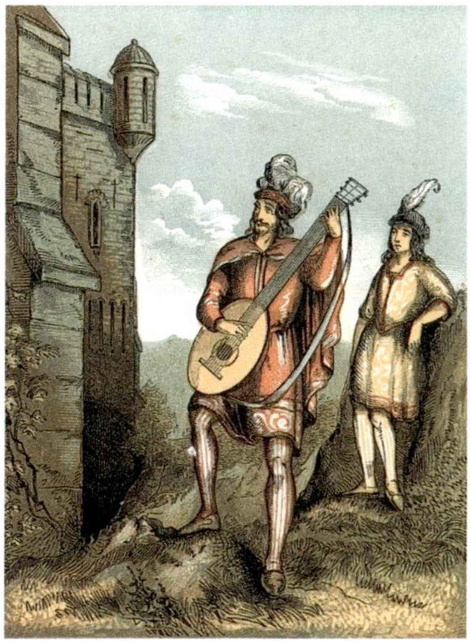

56. Moore, *The Winter Bloom.* Color-printed wood engraving.

Another unusual sideshow in color plate illustration was the printing industry that developed in Rochester, New York, in the 1850s. The booming nursery business of that city needed color plates to illustrate the fruits and plants for sale there. The first plates, produced by stencil and hand coloring by firms such as Sargent (item 70), are perhaps closer to folk art than color printing. These plates were seldom issued as books in editions, but were usually gathered up to suit the individual interests of a customer. As a result, almost all of the Rochester catalogues are unique in their collations. Stencil and hand coloring was eclipsed by chromolithography by the 1870s.

After 1870, full-fledged chromolithography, using ever more complex methods, multiple stones, and overprintings, was the primary medium of color book illustration until the end of the century. Its foremost practitioner, Louis Prang, brought the art to its highest level (see items 66, 96, 99, 102, 103). In Prang's final works, as many as thirty-nine stones were used to extraordinary effect.

The technology of photography began to enter the printing industry in the 1850s. The first color plate book to use photolithography, *Villas on the Hudson* (item 62), appeared in 1860. Its two tones of color were applied over a tinted photolithograph. Most early photolithography was uncolored, and there are few examples that qualify as color plate books. The melding of color and photography is rare before 1890. By 1889, such processes as a heliochrome were used in Whitefield's *The Homes of Our Forefathers* (item 109). However, the printing industry after the Civil War rapidly became more sophisticated in the creation of half-tones, electrotypes, and color printing of all sorts, as seen in two important printers' handbooks: *Harpel's Typograph* (item 92) and Earhart's *The Color Printer* (item 111). These volumes illustrate the extraordinary development of

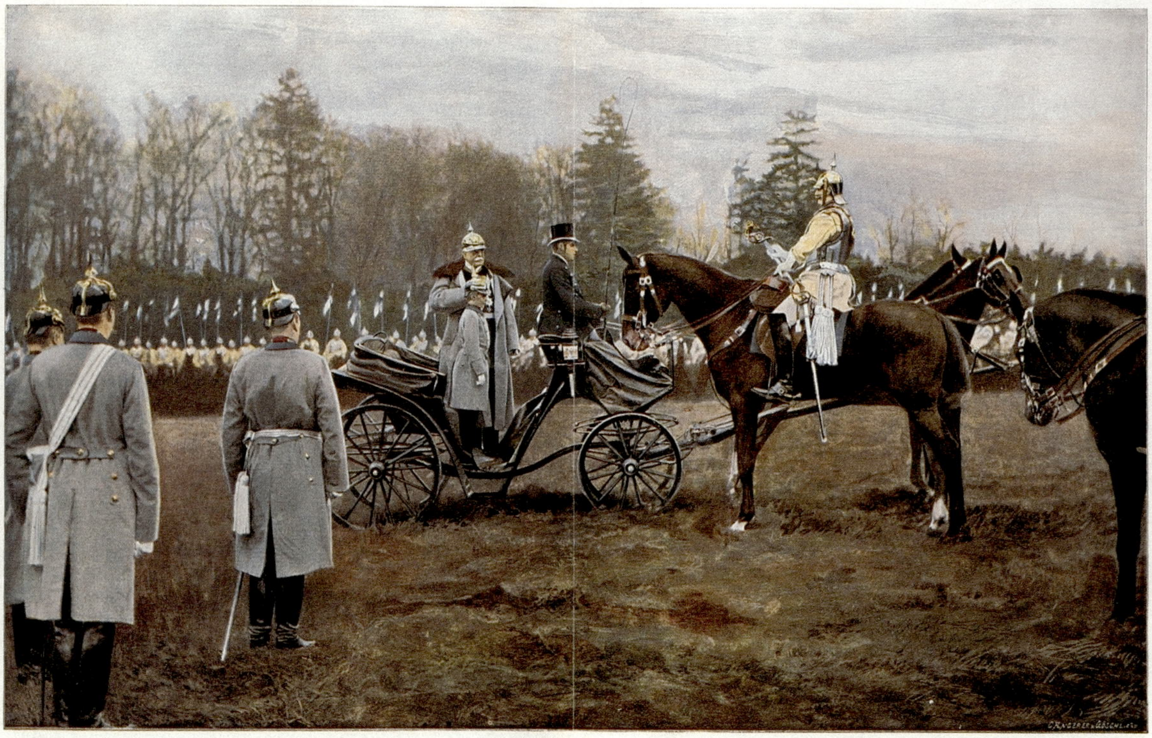

112. Mennell and Garlepp, *Bismarck Denkmal....* Trichromatic half-tone.

color printing skills in the United States from the 1860s to the end of the century. Prior to the 1890s, however, this vast array of color job printing seldom appeared in the form of color plate book illustration, which continued to rely almost exclusively on chromolithography.

In the early 1890s, the marriage of the three-color printing process (fully developed by the time of Earhart's book in 1892) and the photographic half-tone, opened the way to the production of color plates at a fraction of the cost of chromolithography. While the first attempts at this, such as the plates in Mennell's *Bismarck* in 1895 (item 112), were crude compared to the glorious chromolithography Prang was producing at the same time, the cost effectiveness of the new medium was the deciding factor. The end of the century saw the first trickle of books illustrated with trichromatic half-tones, a process which soon drove chromolithography from the field. With advances in printing skills and the addition of black to the mix of the three primary colors, it emerged in the early 20th century as the four-color process, the dominant technology in color printing until the digital revolution of modern times. Thus the end of the 19th century also saw the effective end of the forms of color plate production which had served artists, printers, and publishers through the first hundred years of American color plate books.

Themes in Color Plate Books

This exhibition is organized along broad chronological and generic themes that attempt to emphasize the different kinds of subjects addressed by color plate books and how they evolved through the century. While a myriad of topics were taken as the subjects for illustration with color plates, some broad generalizations can be made about the prevailing themes in American color plate books.

The single most important area of color plate illustration was in the field of natural history. From Alexander Wilson's *American Ornithology* onward, books which described the flora and fauna of the United States were lavishly produced and sold well. While there were a few failures, many of these projects, in spite of being quite large and expensive by the standards of their times, were successfully carried to completion and, in a number of cases, warranted reprinting or new, revised, editions. If we were to take the hundred largest color plate books issued during the century, purely on the basis of the number and size of the plates, the majority of them would be works of natural history.

Natural history books were produced throughout the century, but the golden age of these works fell between 1820 and 1860. This period saw the original publications of all the Audubon works, as well as those of Barton, Bigelow, Say, Holbrook, Michaux, Nuttall, Carson, and Hovey. The most important government publications with major natural history components, such as the "Natural History of New York" series, the Pacific Railroad Surveys, and other explorations of the American West, all appeared in these years as well (see cases 2, 4, and 7).

After 1870 there was a sharp decline in the publication of color plate natural history works. A primary reason may have been the increasingly technical nature of such publications, which were no longer produced by artist-naturalists, but by scientists more interested in precision, even if rendered in black and white.

The major publications of the first several decades of the century were large view books. As already noted, this wonderful genre never caught hold in the United States, and there are relatively few large-format examples. Nonetheless, those that do exist, such as the *Hudson River Portfolio* and *The Yellowstone National Park*, are among the most important American color plate books. The dearth of American view books is countered to some extent by the many topographical plates which appear in the government survey publications (see cases 1, 7, and 9).

Gift books, literary annuals, and similar works, which I have collectively called the "literature of sentiment," account for a great many American color plate books, although generally on a small scale. These genres were at the height of their popularity from 1830 to 1860, although examples can be found throughout the century. Most of the fictional works with color plates are stories found in the annuals. The plates in these books vary widely, from decorative botanical plates to imitations of illuminated manuscripts. The common theme is the desire for a decorative and more or less elaborate presentation, and their bindings often outshine the plates within (see cases 5 and 8).

Works on costume and fashion appeared throughout the century. Fashion plates, as has been noted, were produced in profusion, but almost entirely for periodicals. The handful of fashion books depended heavily on European works. A more consistent illustration of native American fashion is found in the military costume books, which began with *The Soldier's Manual* in 1824 (item 46) and continued for the rest of the century. The majority of these were issued by the government after the Civil War. Works showing typical fashions of a place or race of people, that had been so popular in Europe, found little favor in the United States. The two most notable examples are shown here, Fremaux's *New Orleans Characters* (item 93) and Van Lennup's *The Oriental Album* (item 97).

The depiction of Native Americans was a theme which was consistently interesting to American audiences. It prompted several of the best works of the century, including those of McKenney and Hall and the American edition of Catlin. It was also a consistent element in the many government reports on the American West, as well as many personal narratives (see case 3).

Medical books, which often required color to accurately illustrate diseases or surgical techniques, have largely been ignored by the traditional bibliographers of American color plate books. This seems to be largely on the grounds that the plates are not decorative, or are indeed downright distasteful. This is unfortunate, because there is a large and varied medical literature employing color plates. A representative group is shown here (items 77 through 81, case 7).

Another area neglected by such students as Whitman Bennett is architecture. Here the subject matter can hardly be deemed offensive. From the early 1850s onward there appeared a wealth of architecture and interior design books with color plates, designed to introduce an increasingly affluent American audience to "good taste" in home building and furnishing, as well as the design and landscaping of grounds (see case 6).

Science, in the form of medicine and natural history, had employed color plates almost from the beginning of the century. Beginning about 1840, color plates began to be used in publications in a variety of emerging scientific fields such as geology and chemistry, or the display of quantitative information. Once again, many of these plates appeared in government sponsored works (see case 7).

Not surprisingly, the printing trades produced a number of reference works on color printing illustrated with color plates. Such printers as Harpel, Earhart, and Prang all produced instructional and sample books which are masterpieces of the art they practiced. In the 1880s artists' books began to appear, such as Howard Pyle's illustrated version of *The Lady of Shalott* (item 95). Color plates also began to illustrate large works of art history, most notably the catalogue of the Walters collection of oriental ceramics (item 103). The last quarter of the century brought an increased emphasis on artists and the arts in American color plate books (see cases 8 and 9).

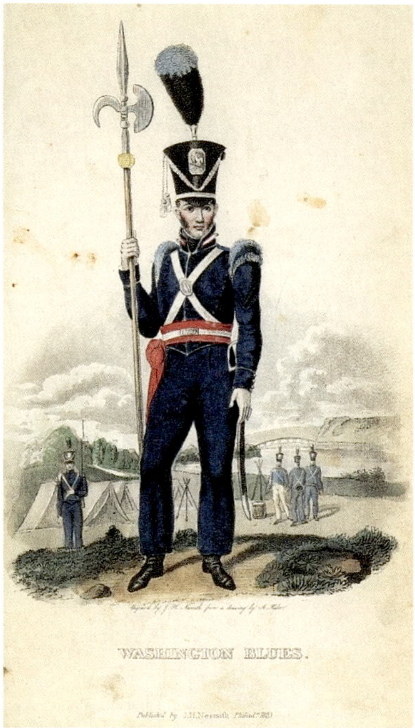

46. [Pennsylvania Militia], *The Soldier's Manual....* Hand-colored copper plate engraving.

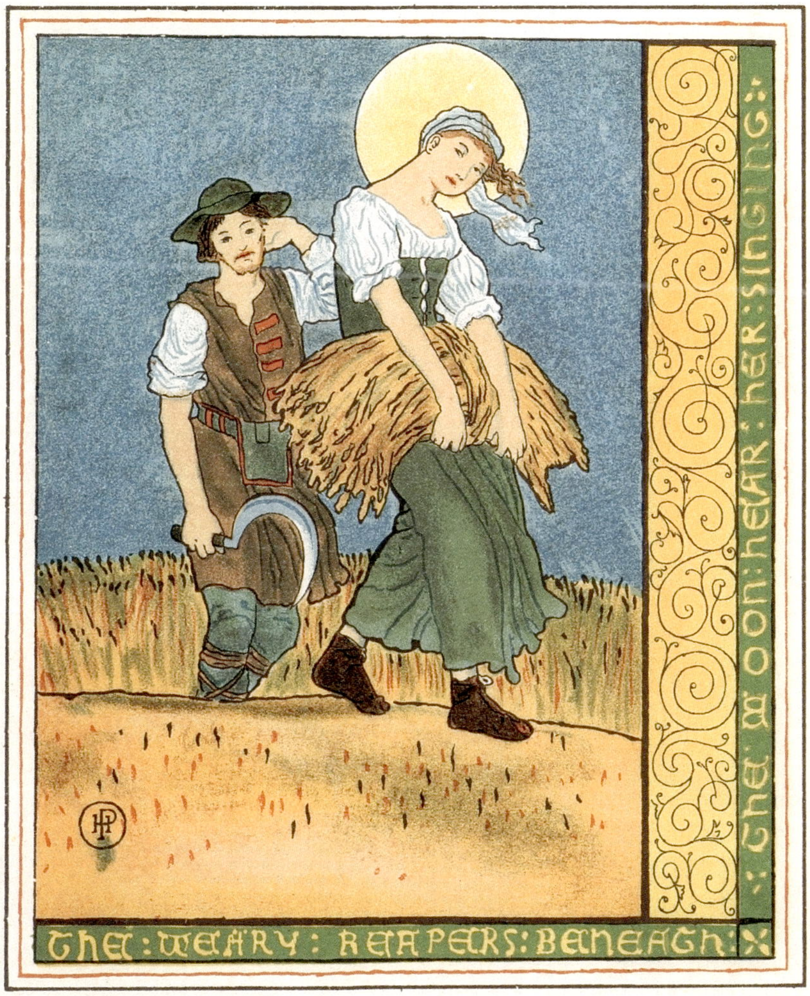

95. Tennyson,
The Lady of Shalott. . . .
Chromotypograph.

The list of American color plate genres can go on and on, although the major types have been delineated above. There are popular histories with crude woodcuts, manuals of flags and signals, guides to currency and coins, sporting books, comic pieces, works on playing cards, and many more. All add to the interest and variety of American color plate books in the 19th century.

Ten Notable Works

While this exhibition is intended to show the broadest possible range of American color plate books, it is impossible not to single out a few of the most salient titles.

No American color plate books command more superlatives than the works of the Audubon family. John James Audubon originally contemplated American publication of his famous *The Birds of America*, and visited Philadelphia in 1824 for that reason. There he realized that no American printer was capable of executing the work on the scale he envisioned, and that the hostility of some members of the local scientific establishment would make the task impossible. He took his project to England, where the double elephant folio *Birds* was produced in London, in 1826–1839. After its completion, Audubon was anxious to return permanently to the United States. He chose to produce the octavo edition of *The Birds of America* (item 34) in Philadelphia, where the plates were executed by the firm of James T. Bowen between 1840 and 1844, under the close supervision of Audubon and his sons. Although an expensive work, at one hundred dollars a set, it was within the reach of many well-to-do citizens. The octavo *Birds* was good value for the price. With five hundred hand-colored plates, it was the most extensive color plate book produced in America up to that time. The Audubons were effective salesmen, canvassing the country and obtaining hundreds of subscriptions. Ultimately, the octavo *Birds* went through numerous 19th-century editions, both in the hands of the Audubons and later of the New York publisher, Roe, Lockwood. It must be accounted the single most successful color plate project of the century in its scope and market success.

Even while the octavo *Birds* was in press, the Audubons launched *The Viviparous Quadrupeds of North America*, published in elephant folio between 1843 and 1848, and in octavo between 1849 and 1854 (items 36, 37, 38). The folio edition was the largest single color plate book to be carried to a successful conclusion during the century. While the *Quadrupeds* project was probably not as lucrative as the octavo *Birds*, it was commercially viable, and the octavo edition also went through numerous editions. Once again, all of the plates were produced by the Bowen firm.

In 1858, with his father dead, and brother Victor terminally ill, John Woodhouse Audubon made the ill-fated decision to attempt a reprint of the double elephant folio *Birds* in chromolithography. Working with Julius Bien of New York, John Woodhouse had by 1860 published 105 plates, reproducing 150 of the original edition (small images such as warblers were doubled up) (item 40). The advent of the Civil War caused many subscribers to back out, and the immensely expensive project collapsed, consuming the family savings and literally killing John Woodhouse with overwork and worry. The publisher, Roe, Lockwood, was left in possession of all the completed plates and, evidently, the copyrights to all of the family publications. Although only a part of the intended work, and a catastrophe as a publication, the "Bien edition" of the *Birds*, as it is usually called, is the largest and most ambitious color plate book of the century. No other artists or publishers approached the enterprises of the Audubons in the size and extent of the projects they undertook.

After the works of the Audubons, the largest and most successful work was the *History of the Indian Tribes of North America*, usually known as "McKenney and Hall," after Thomas L. McKenney (the Commissioner of Indian Affairs whose idea the book was) and James Hall (the prolific Cincinnati journalist

24. McKenny and Hall,
History of the Indian Tribes....
Hand-colored lithograph.

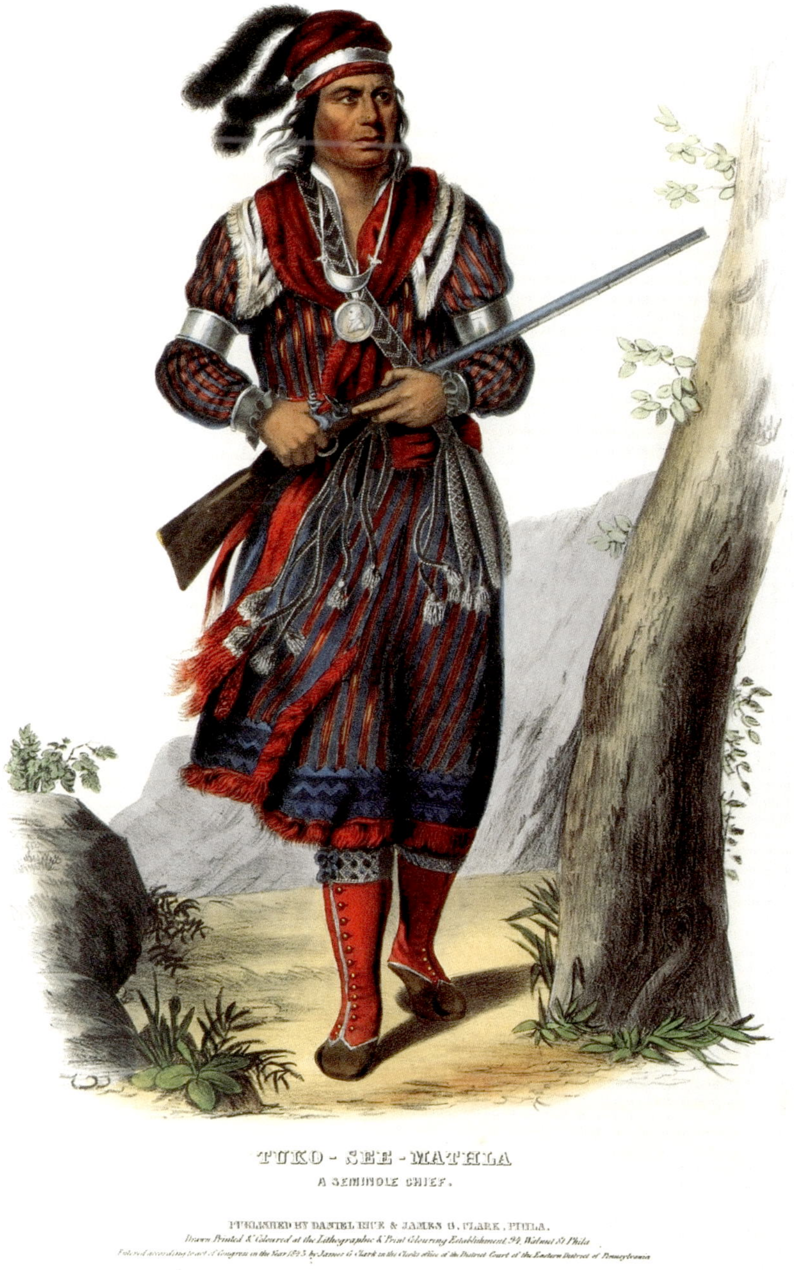

who supplied the text). Neither can claim any responsibility beyond selection for the work's 120 plates, based on portraits of leading chiefs by Charles Bird King and lithographed by the firms of Lehman and Duval, and J. T. Bowen. The folio edition, which was issued in parts between 1836 and 1844 (after years of preliminary toil), was the most ambitious work produced in America prior to those of the Audubons (item 24). McKenney and Hall imitated them in also publishing a more affordable octavo version, which went through multiple editions between 1848 and the 1870s. By the time the final edition appeared, many of the original lithographic stones were lost or worn out, and replacement plates had to be supplied in chromolithography.

Many people consider the *Hudson River Portfolio* to be the greatest American color plate book of the century. One of the few aquatint books published in the United States, it was a collaboration between two recent English immigrants: the engraver, John Hill, and the artist, William Guy Wall. Issued in New York between 1821 and 1825, it is the most ambitious landscape view book in the European tradition undertaken in America (item 6). Its twenty plates, showing views on the Hudson River from the north down to New York Harbor, are extraordinary for their skillful execution and luminous engraving and coloring. It is certainly the foremost American book of its kind.

Another grand American project was the edition of George Catlin's *North American Indian Portfolio* published by the New York lithographer, James Ackerman (item 25). Catlin had originally published his *Portfolio* in London in 1844, but he had nothing to do with the American edition, which was an out-and-out piracy executed without his knowledge or consent. Ackerman not only ignored Catlin's copyright, but undercut the market for the London edition by pricing his edition less expensively, and then used the preface to suggest that Catlin would have done better to publish in New York. His rather cheeky introduction is a manifesto for the American color plate book, and deserves to be quoted in full:

> To the American Public. A young American artist ventures to challenge for his works that encouragement which has hitherto been ministered too sparingly to American productions. As a nation, we have so long been reproached with inability to produce pictorial embellishments equal to the European that, although a mistake, it has become a received opinion.
>
> The enthusiastic author of the London Edition of this splendid and talented work has practically succumbed to the prevailing yet unjust prejudice, and has carried the results of his daring genius and enterprise to a foreign mart; sending from abroad, and from the hands of European artists, an American production in foreign habiliments to be patronized in the author's own land.
>
> The Artist and publisher of the republication on this side of the water, evincing through this, his enterprise, of AMERICAN ART, an abiding confidence in the taste, judgement and liberality of his countrymen, has ventured (with a mere change of dress), to offer a cheaper, and he trusts, a better edition than the costly London copy.

75. [Pacific Railroad Surveys], *Reports of Explorations and Surveys. . . .* Tinted lithograph with hand coloring.

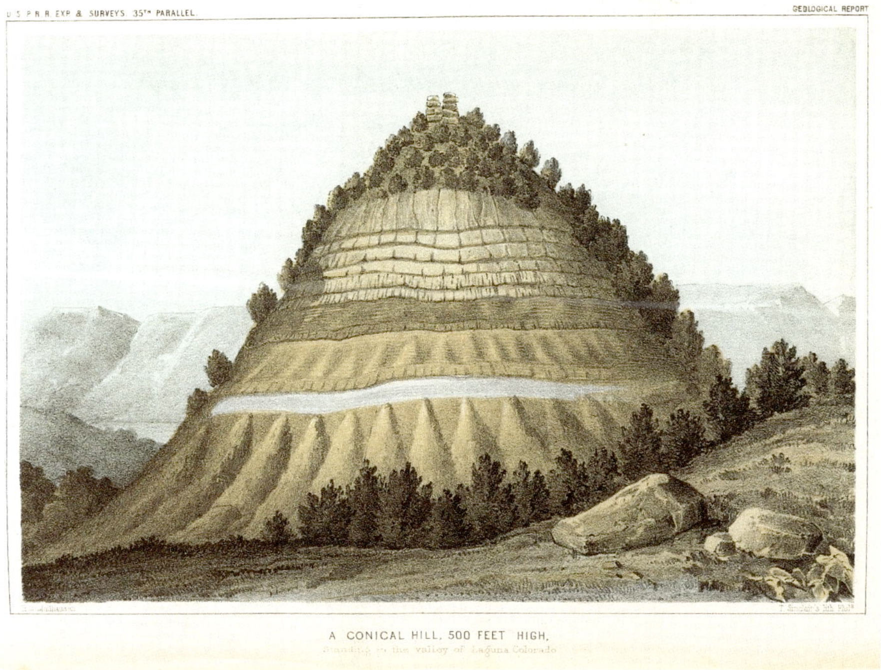

> Fully equal, or greatly superior, the critical justice of the country may decide it to be. Of this favorable result, hope may tell the Artist a 'flattering tale,' yet he would plead enthusiasm, without which the life and spirit of all art dies. At all events, the greater cheapness of this edition is as unquestionable, as that it is purely 'American fabric' recommends its patronage.
>
> In fact, the Artist would contest the received opinion, that nothing pictorial can be executed in this country equal to the European productions, and would leave his countrymen to carry out the experiment, whether it be not that patronage is alone wanting to produce originals – or republications equal if not superior to those of all Europe.
>
> This venture, receiving no impulse from the powerful arm of an overflowing government treasury, starts on an 'Exploring Expedition' of its own, into the waters of criticism; and, if but prosperous gales attend its return, the grateful Artist pledges his unwearied efforts to produce nothing but the best specimens of American delineative art, wherewith to acknowledge the patronage and indulgence of his countrymen and to vindicate the capacity of our native artists. J. A.

Despite this bold pronouncement, the Ackerman edition of Catlin seems to have had only limited success. After Ackerman went out of business, the lithographic stones were purchased by Currier & Ives, who altered the captions and reissued them as individual prints in 1865 (item 26).

Pride of place in American color plate books must always go to William Birch, whose *The City of Philadelphia. . . In the Year 1800* (item 1) was the pioneering work of the genre. An accomplished artist and miniaturist, Birch engraved all of the plates for his collection of street and building scenes. It was a remarkably ambitious work at the time, and only a few small individual color

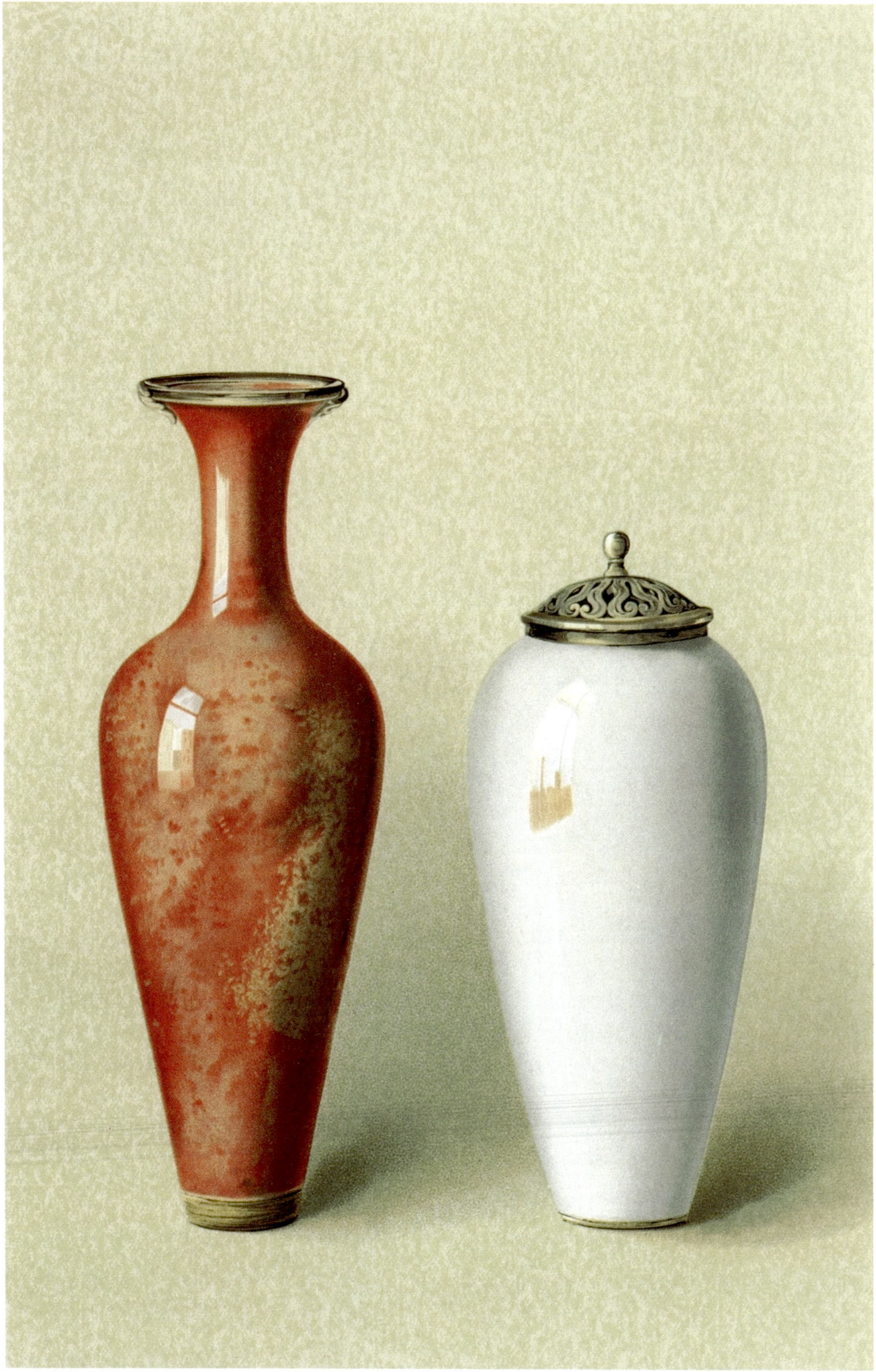

103. Walters and Bushell, *Oriental Ceramic Art. . . .*
Chromolithograph.

plates predate it in American publishing. The book was sufficiently popular for Birch to reissue it in somewhat varying formats in 1804, 1809, and 1828.

Government sponsorship of large publication projects using color plates probably accounted for the printing of more individual plates than all other works combined, both because of the scope of the projects and the number of copies printed. It is estimated that the Pacific Railroad Surveys, with thirteen volumes and print runs of at least ten thousand copies each, required twenty-one million plates, both colored and black and white. The Railroad Surveys is a monument to American illustration unsurpassed in its century, and it exemplifies the acceptance of a governmental role in gathering and lavishly publishing scientific data (item 75).

Lastly, the Boston printer and publisher, Louis Prang, was responsible for the two grandest American books of the age of chromolithography. His plates for Ferdinand V. Hayden's *The Yellowstone National Park* (item 99), based on originals by Thomas Moran, were the first American book illustrations to fully realize the potentials of chromolithography. Prang, the greatest chromolithographer in the United States, dominated his field for the last quarter of the 19th century and spearheaded its technical advance. He was arguably the first color printer in America to carry his craft beyond anything done in Europe. His final book, the catalogue of the great Walters collection of oriental porcelain (item 103), was his finest achievement and the apogee of American chromolithography.

While the ten works cited above are among the most significant 19th-century American color plate books, the field does not lend itself to "best books" lists. Some small books have charms greater than the major works, while others are notable triumphs of craftsmanship on a modest scale. This exhibition, while displaying many of the highlights of the century, aims to show the diversity of color plate work as well as these leading titles. While many of the books would be on any list of the most interesting, others simply represent the kinds of books in which color plates commonly appeared. In sum, they provide the viewer with an insight into the tastes and interests of the 19th century and, in parallel, the evolution of the techniques of production which created the color plate book in America.

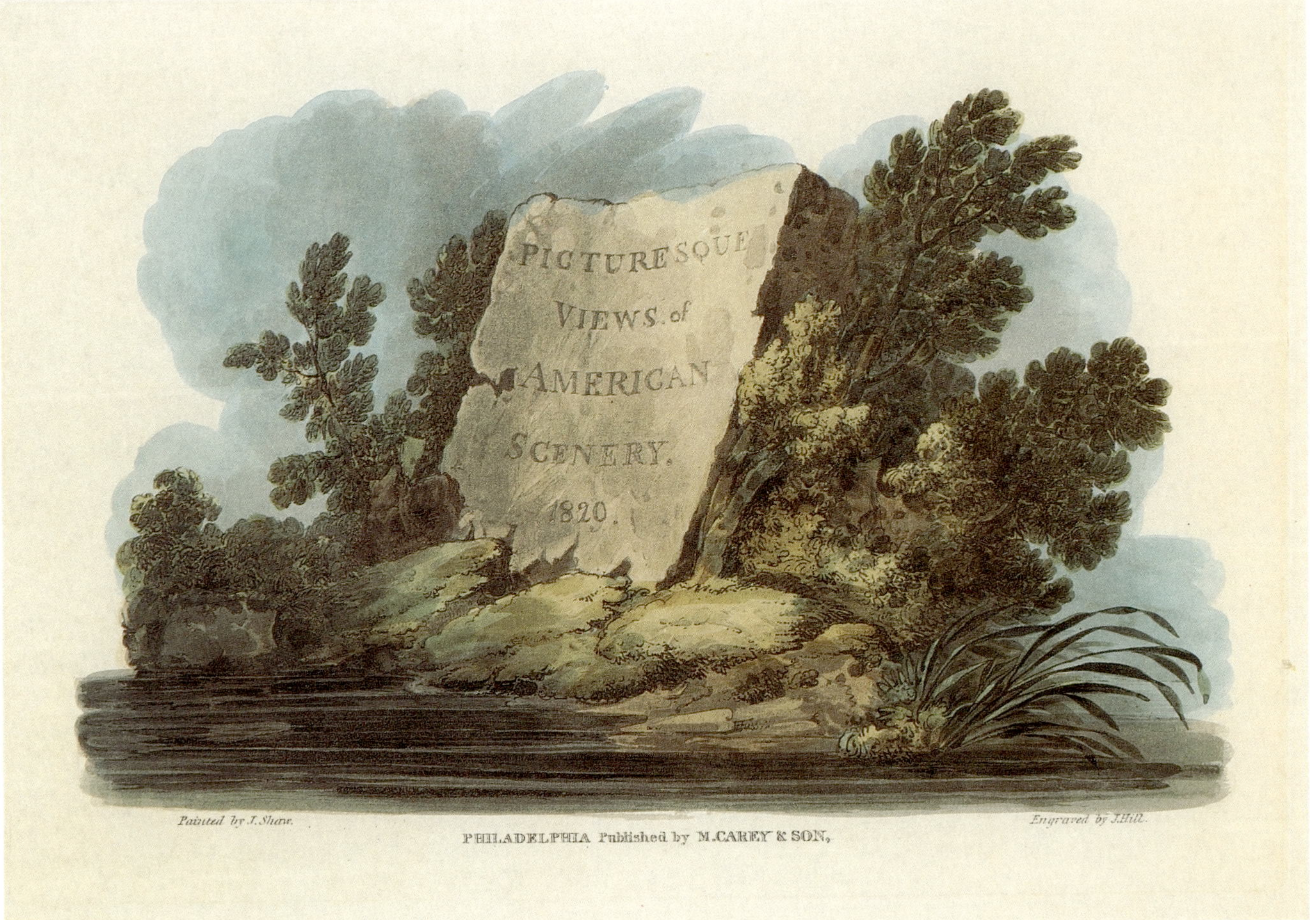

5. Shaw and Hill, *Picturesque Views, of American Scenery....*
Aquatint with hand coloring.

CASE I: Beginnings 1800–1825

American color plate books had a fitful beginning in the first quarter of the 19th century. The best works of the period, the landscape view books, all issued in parts, uniformly failed to retain subscribers long enough to meet their original projected size. Despite a brilliant start with William Birch's two books in 1800 and 1808, and the individual achievements of John Hill, whose aquatints are among the finest of American color plates, there were few successful publications. There was a limited audience sufficiently affluent to support the high cost of labor and printing involved in producing color plate books. The works that were accomplished were heavily dependent on the talents of immigrant European craftsmen, for few Americans possessed the necessary skills. Despite these drawbacks, some books of extraordinary quality were produced.

1. William R. Birch: *The City of Philadelphia, in the State of Pennsylvania North America: as it Appeared in the Year 1800....* Springland, Pa.: W. Birch, 1800.

Hand-colored copper plate engraving

The color plate book in America sprang full blown upon the stage with the publication of this work, conceived and published by the painter and engraver, William Birch. Having immigrated from England in 1794, he offered a patriotic justification for his project, hoping it was a vehicle "by which the improvements of the country could be conveyed to Europe." The twenty-eight plates showed every aspect of life in the burgeoning city in richly detailed images, displaying aspects of architecture, commerce, fashion, trade, and daily life. Despite the high price ($44.50, bound and colored), there were about 150 initial subscribers. There was sufficient interest in the work to allow Birch to reissue it in variant formats in 1804, 1809, and 1828.

2. William R. Birch: *The Country Seats of the United States of North America, with Some Scenes Connected with Them.* Springland, near Bristol, Pa.: Designed and published by W. B., enamel painter, 1808.

Hand-colored copper plate engraving

Birch's skill as a miniaturist is demonstrated in his charming second book. Birch and his sons, Thomas and George, collaborated on the work, combining line and stipple engraving with delicate coloring to rich effect. The conception of *Country Seats* was primarily decorative, a handsome series of views aimed at an audience such as might possess country estates themselves. This kind of luxury view book, a genre of immense popularity in England and Europe, never really took hold in the United States. Americans preferred to buy individual views and prints which were produced in huge numbers, but not expensive books.

3. Alexander Wilson: *American Ornithology, or, the Natural History of the Birds of the United States: Illustrated with Plates; Engraved and Colored from Original Drawings Taken from Nature....* Philadelphia: Bradford & Inskeep, 1808–1814.

Hand-colored copper plate engraving

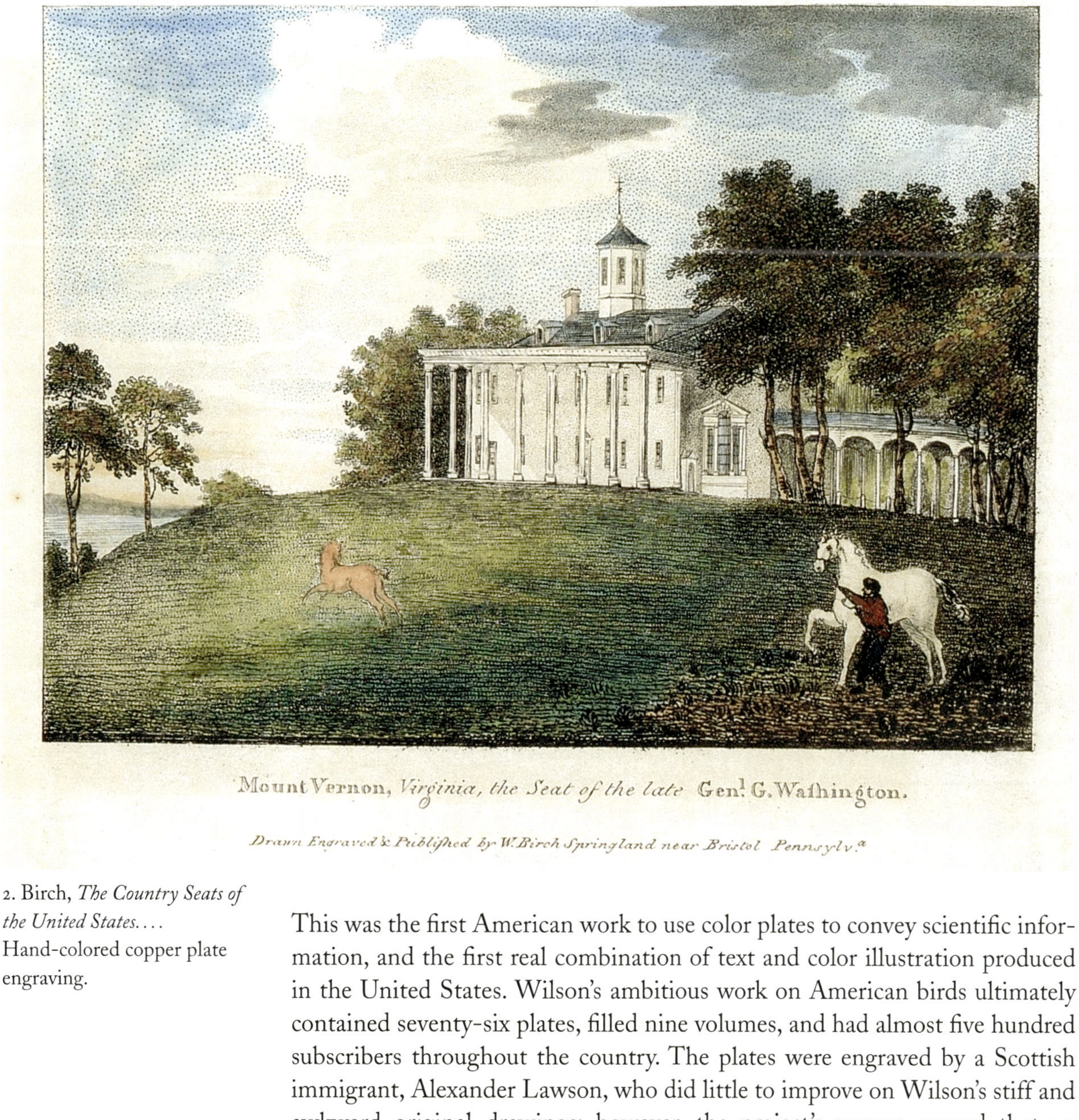

2. Birch, *The Country Seats of the United States. . . .* Hand-colored copper plate engraving.

This was the first American work to use color plates to convey scientific information, and the first real combination of text and color illustration produced in the United States. Wilson's ambitious work on American birds ultimately contained seventy-six plates, filled nine volumes, and had almost five hundred subscribers throughout the country. The plates were engraved by a Scottish immigrant, Alexander Lawson, who did little to improve on Wilson's stiff and awkward original drawings; however, the project's success proved that an American audience would support such a large undertaking. Works of natural history and science, with a concrete function, proved to be more commercially viable in America than luxury works such as view books.

4. Alexander Wilson: *Original Copper Plate for* American Ornithology. Philadelphia: Alexander Lawson, [1811].

Original copper plate

Few original copper plates used in 19th-century book production survive today. They wore down quickly in use, and the value of the metal caused most to be recycled. Some of the plates for Wilson's work do survive, although probably reworked for the second American edition of 1829, which employed the same plates. The engraved figures appear in mirror image to the final print.

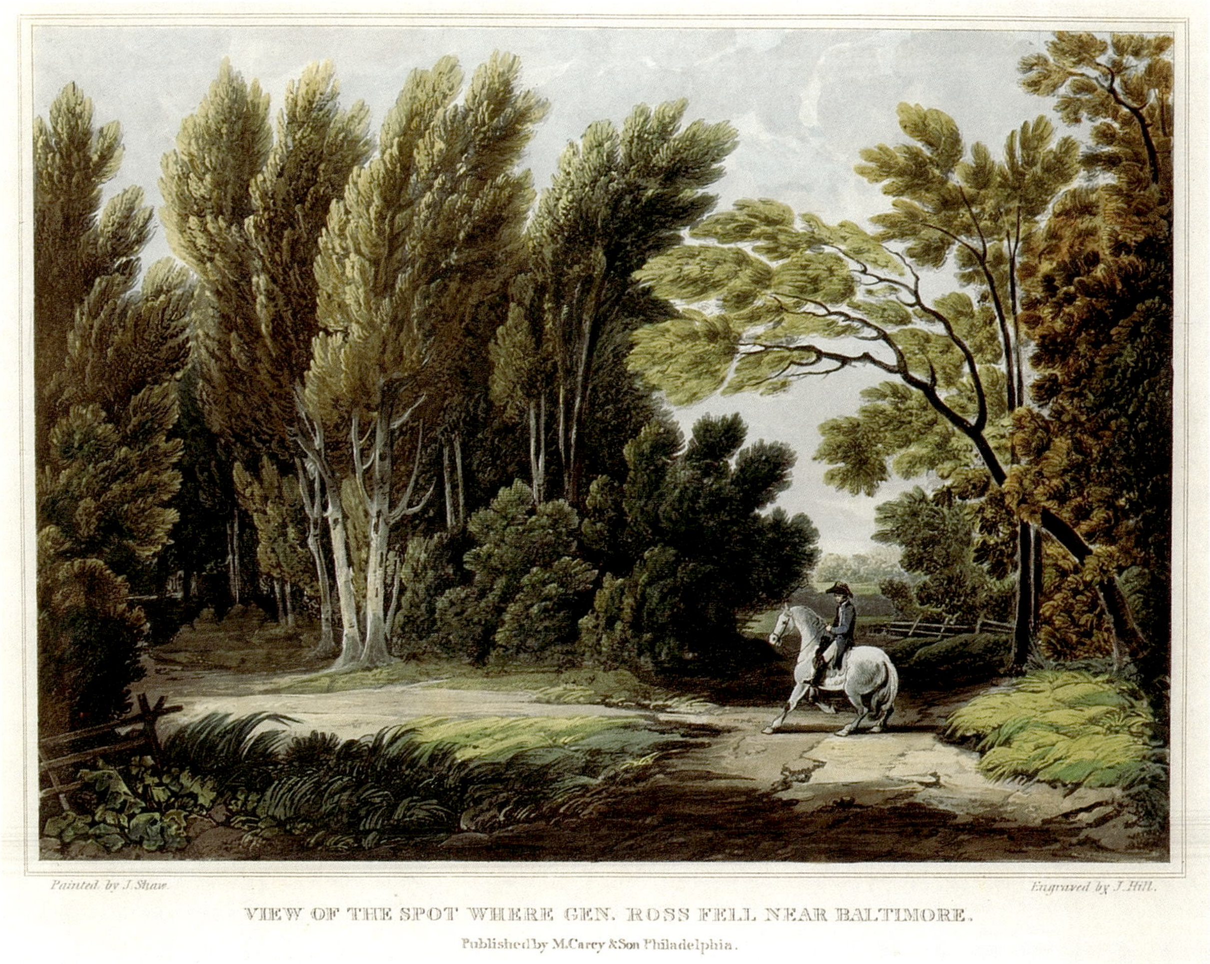

5. Shaw and Hill, *Picturesque Views, of American Scenery....* Aquatint with hand coloring.

5. [Joshua Shaw and John Hill]: *Picturesque Views, of American Scenery, 1819. Painted by J. Shaw. Engraved by J. Hill.* Philadelphia: Published by Moses Thomas, [1819].

Aquatint with hand coloring

Known as "The Landscape Album," this portfolio of views was a collaboration between the artist, Joshua Shaw, and the aquatint engraver, John Hill. The latter had only just arrived from England when he began work on the project. It was proposed as a work celebrating "the best and most popular Views" in America, since "Our country abounds with Scenery, comprehending all the varieties of the sublime, the beautiful, and the picturesque in nature, worthy to engage the skill of an Artist...." Six parts of six plates each were originally proposed, but only half were issued before the project foundered because of a lack of subscribers.

Time and again, ambitious projects such as this, issued in parts, collapsed before reaching completion. The failure of these publications illustrates the thinness of the market for such expensive works in America.

6. William G. Wall: *The Hudson River Portfolio.* [New York: Henry G. Megarey, 1821–1825].

Aquatint with hand coloring

This grand book, the collaboration of two English immigrants to the United States, is often considered the finest American color plate book of the 19th century. As with so many other important ventures in color in America, it owed its quality to foreign training. The twenty plates, based on originals by William Guy Wall and engraved in aquatint by John Hill, trace the course of the Hudson River from north to south, concluding with a view of New York harbor. Sadly, it is almost an anomaly in form and medium; it is one of very few aquatint works produced in the United States during a brief florescence in the 1820s, and one of a handful of folio view books published in America.

7. Fielding Lucas: *The Art of Drawing, Colouring and Painting Landscapes, in Water Colours Accompanied with Ten Engravings.* Baltimore: Fielding Lucas, 1815.

Aquatint with hand coloring

Fielding Lucas was perhaps the most successful American publisher of 1810–1830, following the path of Benjamin Franklin and Isaiah Thomas in building a distribution network for his books throughout the United States. He was also one of the first to experiment with color illustration in books outside of the large works issued by subscription, such as Birch or Wilson. Lucas clearly saw that the addition of color could be an effective marketing tool for publishers. This book of drawing instruction is the first American example of a popular genre.

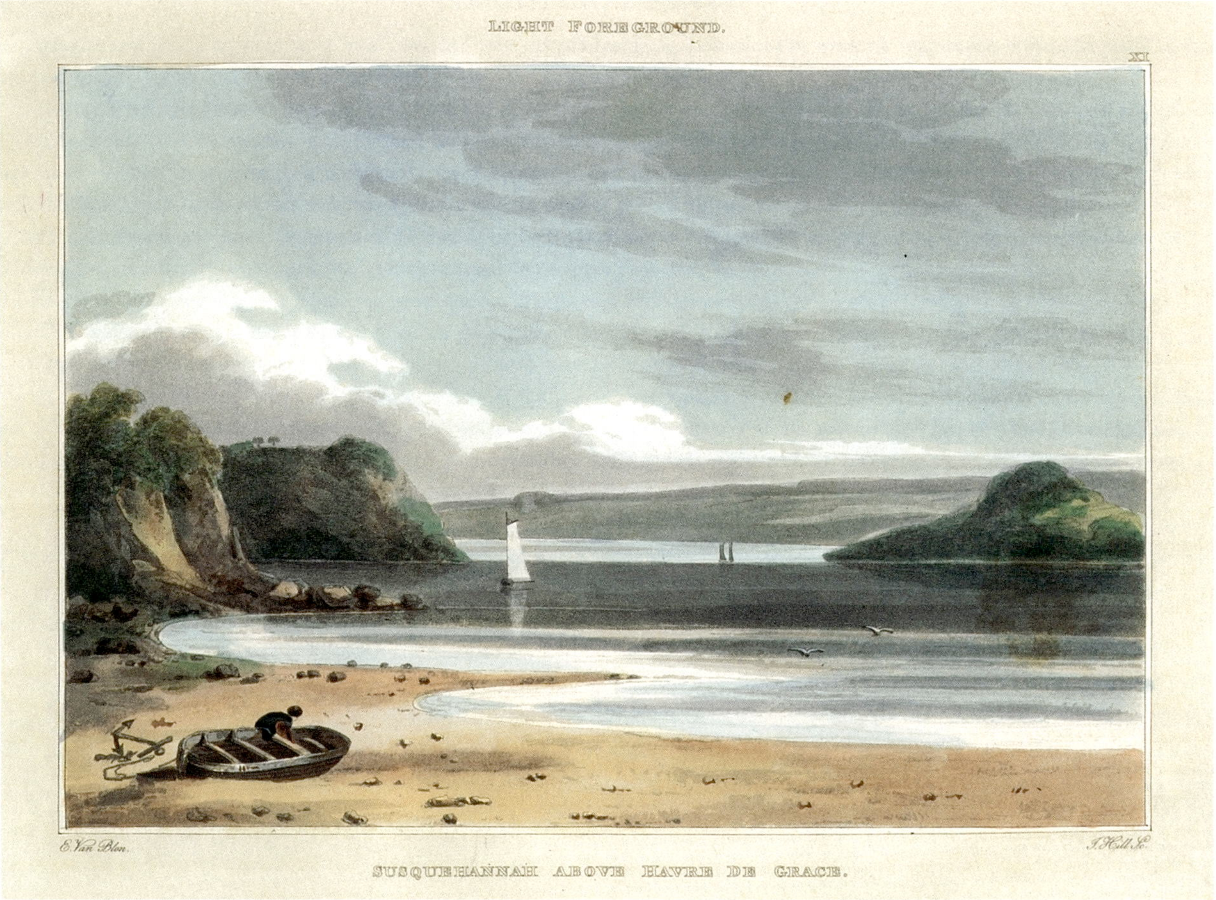

8. Lucas,
Progressive Drawing Book. . . .
Aquatint with hand coloring.

8. Fielding Lucas: *Lucas' Progressive Drawing Book, in Three Parts . . . Consisting Chiefly of Original Views of American Scenery, and Embracing the Latest and Best Improvements in the Mode of Instruction.* Baltimore: Fielding Lucas, 1827.

Aquatint with hand coloring

The most ambitious of Lucas' publications, with drawing instruction and landscape views by John H. B. Latrobe, executed in aquatint by John Hill. Lucas freely confessed to having borrowed heavily from English works on drawing in compiling the book, but he sought as much as possible to use American views in order "to stamp it with national character." In this case, Lucas was producing a book which would compete in the marketplace with imported English works, and he probably hoped to capitalize on the patriotic element lent by the American scenes.

9. [William Combe]: *The Tour of Dr. Syntax in Search of the Picturesque.* Philadelphia: Published and sold by W. Charles, [ca. 1819].

Aquatint with hand coloring

This pirated American edition of William Combe's popular satire is a close copy of the English original, including the thirty-one aquatint plates. William Charles, another immigrant from Scotland, spent much of his career in New York and Philadelphia, cheerfully knocking off English satirical prints for an American audience. He acted as both engraver and publisher of this book, doing a passable job of imitating Rowlandson. The work was successful enough for Carey & Lea to pirate the *Second Tour* in 1822, after Charles' death.

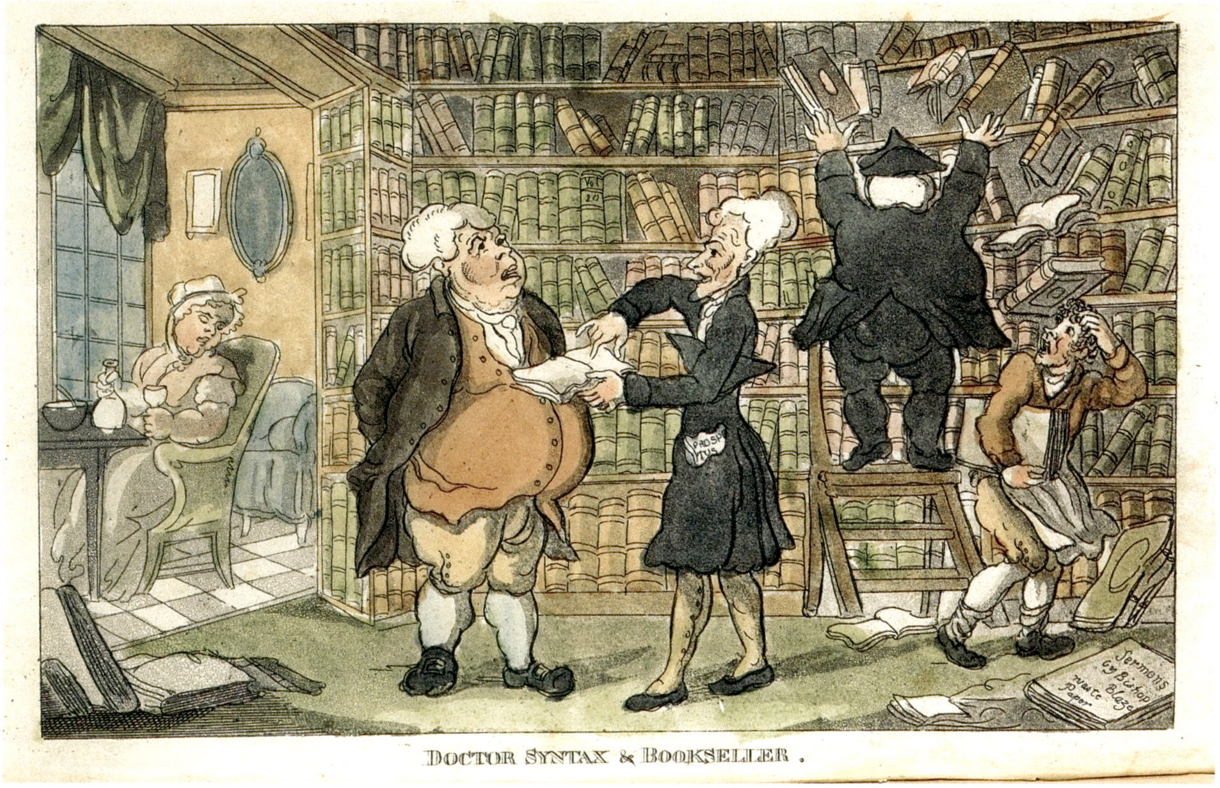

9. Combe,
The Tour of Dr. Syntax. . . .
Aquatint with hand coloring.

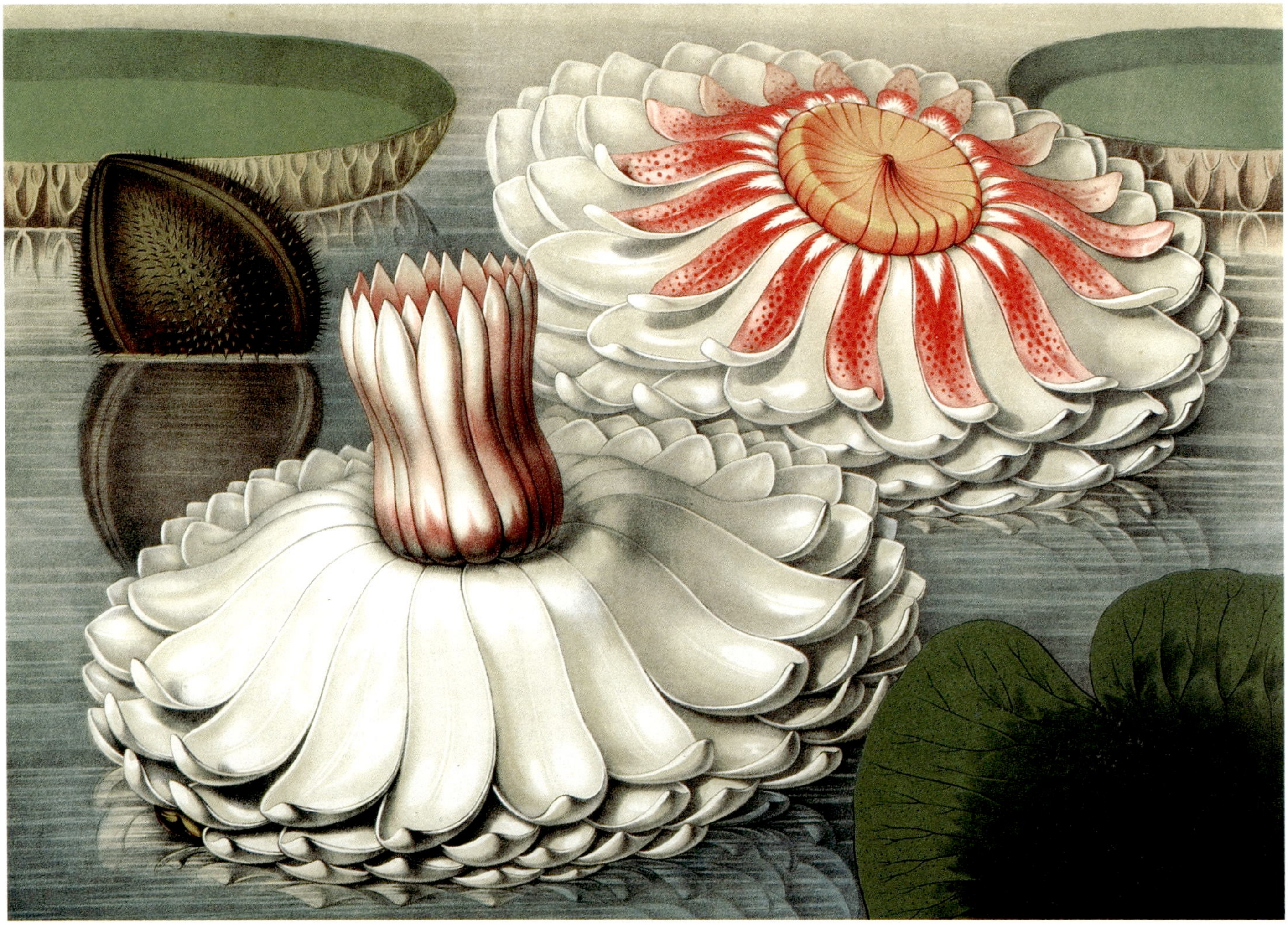

19. Allen, *Victoria Regia*. . . .
Chromolithograph.

CASE 2: The Study of Nature 1817–1857

Natural history studies were the most important area of American color plate book production in the period before the Civil War. Describing American plants and animals, classifying *materia medica,* and cataloging native fruits and flowers accounted for the bulk of major color plate books. Color played a vital role in accurately depicting natural history subjects, essential in creating a full and accurate description of individual species. These topics seemed to find a ready audience to support them by subscription, and some, such as the works of Michaux and Nuttall on American trees, were reprinted many times. Practical interest and national pride combined to make such books viable commercial productions, and some were landmarks in the beginnings of systematic scientific publication in the United States.

10. Jacob Bigelow: *American Medical Botany, Being a Collection of the Native Medicinal Plants of the United States. . . .* Boston: Published by Cummings and Hilliard, 1817–1820.

Color-printed *a la poupée* from etched stone

This is the first botanical work published in America. Bigelow originally planned to use hand-colored copper plate engravings, which are employed in the first half of the first volume. This method proving too expensive and laborious, he sought a method of printing color rather than applying it by hand. Richard Wolfe, who has made an exhaustive study of the work, believes that the rest of the plates (the book was issued in six parts over a three-year period) were made by etching a stone block, then applying the colors to the stone *a la poupée*. The stone, inked with multiple colors, was then printed in a single impression. This is the only use of such a process in an American color plate book.

11. William P. C. Barton: *A Flora of North America, Illustrated by Coloured Figures Drawn from Nature.* Philadelphia: Carey & Lea, 1821–1823.

Stipple engraving with printed color and hand coloring

Barton, the most distinguished botanist in the United States, clearly hoped the plates in the first American flora would match European standards: "It is confidently believed by the author, that they will be found the most successful attempts at imitation, by SOUND engraving, of the French style, yet made in this country." The plates were made by Cornelius Tiebout, the first really skilled engraver born in the United States, although he trained in London for two years in the 1790s to perfect his technique. The plates were partly printed in color and then finished by hand.

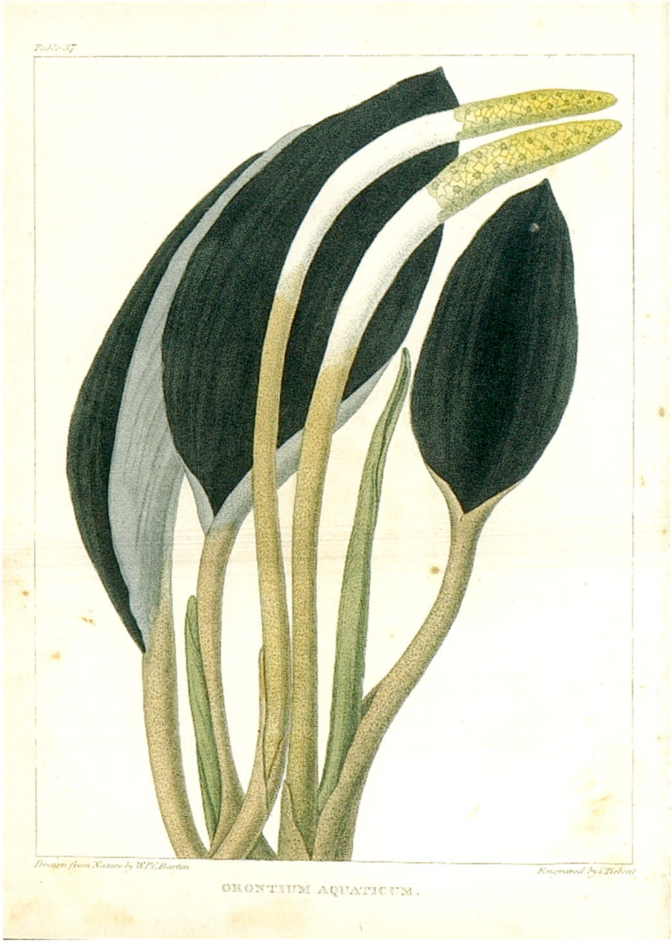

12. Doughty, *The Cabinet of Natural History. . . .* Hand-colored lithograph.

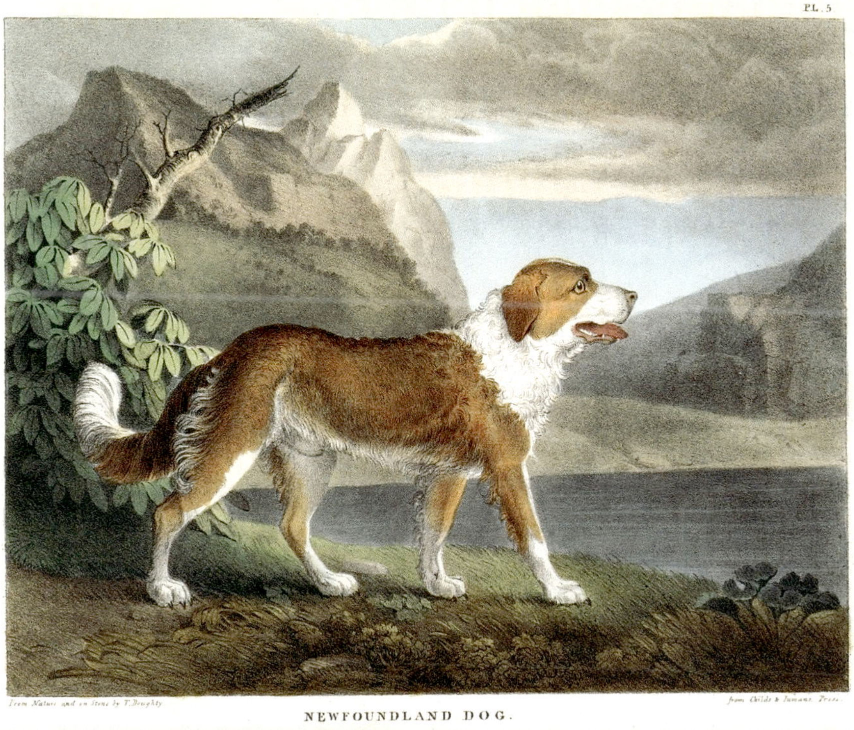

11. Barton, *A Flora of North America. . . .* Stipple engraving with printed color and hand coloring.

12. [John and Thomas Doughty]: *The Cabinet of Natural History, and American Rural Sports with Illustration. . . .* Philadelphia: J. & T. Doughty, 1830–1833.

Hand-colored lithograph

The Doughtys' *Cabinet* is an odd amalgam of natural history, sporting accounts, travel narratives, and practical advice for the countryman. This was the first major book issued in the United States to be illustrated with hand-colored lithographic plates, preceded only by three minor books in the 1820s. It marks the beginning of the dominance of lithography in book illustration, although the process had been commercially viable in America for a decade. The plates in the first volume are by Thomas Doughty, well known as a Hudson River School painter, who executed the drawings on the lithographic stones. *The Cabinet* was issued in monthly numbers, and the plates were undoubtedly designed as an inducement to subscription.

13. Thomas Say: *American Conchology, or Descriptions of the Shells of North America. Illustrated by Coloured Figures from Original Drawings Executed from Nature.* New Harmony, In.: Printed at the School Press, 1830–1838.

Hand-colored copper plate engraving

One of the most exotic American natural history and color plate books, this was produced under frontier conditions in the utopian community of New Harmony, Indiana. Thomas Say, whose *American Entomology* had appeared with notable color plates in Philadelphia between 1824 and 1828, was one of the scientists who moved to this frontier social experiment, funded by Robert Owen, in 1827. This study of American shells was printed on the School Press there, and some of the copper plates were produced there as well (others were brought from Philadelphia). Legend has it that the New Harmony school children aided Mrs. Say in coloring the plates.

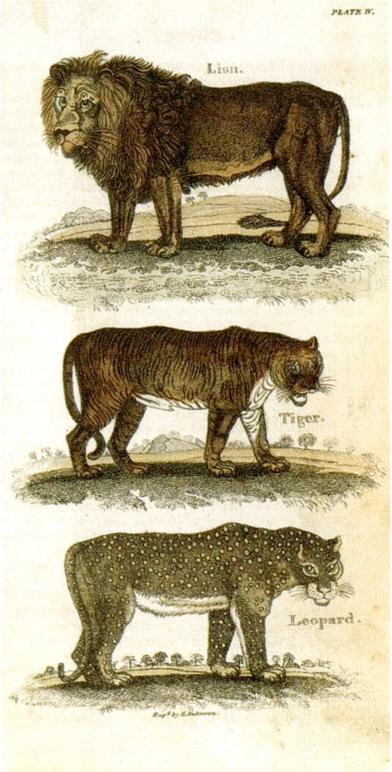

14. Turnbull,
History of Animals....
Hand-colored copper plate engraving.

14. John Turnbull: *History of Animals, Being a Comprehensive Selection from Goldsmith's Animated Nature, with Anecdotes of Animals. Illustrative of their Habits and Characters. Embellished with Twelve Pages of Copperplate Engravings.* Steubenville, Ohio: Published by J. & B. Turnbull, 1831.

Hand-colored copper plate engraving

A modest book, its text entirely lifted from Goldsmith (who lifted it from Buffon), this is one of the first color plate books to be produced west of the Atlantic seaboard. Its engravings were made by Hugh Anderson, who had worked in Philadelphia and then for Fielding Lucas in Baltimore, before moving to Ohio in 1826. Only two complete copies are known to survive.

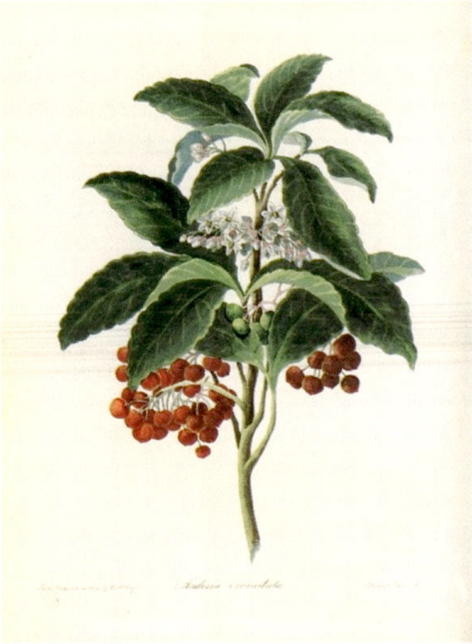
15. Landreth,
The Floral Magazine....
Hand-colored lithograph.

15. D. & C. Landreth: *The Floral Magazine and Botanical Repository, Vol. I....* Philadelphia: D. & C. Landreth, 1832.

Hand-colored lithograph

The Landreth nursery was one of the oldest in the United States. This volume, the only one they published, was probably issued partly as a promotion for the Landreth business and partly as a contribution to botanical knowledge. The thirty plates were printed and colored by four different Philadelphia lithographers and show considerable variation in quality. Evidently the Landreths contracted out the color work almost plate by plate. Excepting a few productions such as this in Philadelphia, it was not until the late 1850s that nurseries began to extensively publish plates of flowers to promote sales.

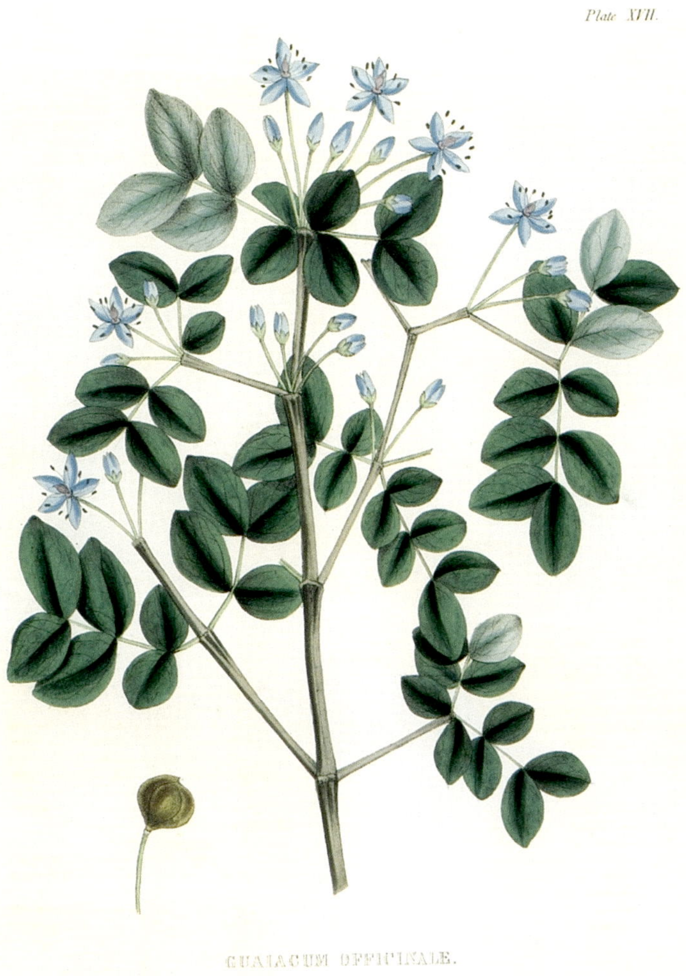

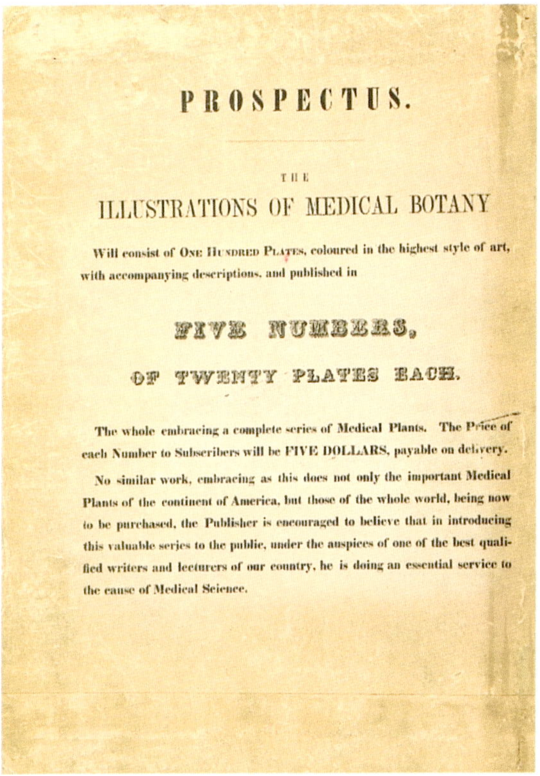

PROSPECTUS.

THE

ILLUSTRATIONS OF MEDICAL BOTANY

Will consist of ONE HUNDRED PLATES, coloured in the highest style of art, with accompanying descriptions, and published in

FIVE NUMBERS,

OF TWENTY PLATES EACH.

The whole embracing a complete series of Medical Plants. The Price of each Number to Subscribers will be FIVE DOLLARS, payable on delivery.

No similar work, embracing as this does not only the important Medical Plants of the continent of America, but those of the whole world, being now to be purchased, the Publisher is encouraged to believe that in introducing this valuable series to the public, under the auspices of one of the best qualified writers and lecturers of our country, he is doing an essential service to the cause of Medical Science.

16. Carson, *Illustrations of Medical Botany. . . .* Hand-colored lithograph.

16. Joseph Carson: *Illustrations of Medical Botany: Consisting of Coloured Figures of the Plants, Affording the Most Important Articles of the Materia Medica.* Philadelphia: Robert P. Smith, 1847.

Hand-colored lithograph

The most elaborate of work of medical botany was that of Dr. Joseph Carson of Philadelphia, illustrated with one hundred hand-colored lithographs heightened with gum arabic. As with most of the large color plate projects of this period, it was issued in parts. Robert P. Smith was also the publisher of the works of Michaux and Nuttall on American trees.

17. Morris Mattson: *The American Vegetable Practice, or a New and Improved Guide to Health, Designed for the Use of Families....* Boston: Published by Daniel L. Hale, 1841.

Chromolithograph

Mattson's *materia medica* is the first American book with plates printed by chromolithography. All of the color is printed, and none is applied by hand. A separate pull of the plate was required to apply each separate color, with up to five colors appearing in some plates, and occasional more elaborate effects created by overprinting. William Sharp, an English printer who had recently immigrated to Boston, produced the plates. He had experimented in chromolithography during his apprenticeship in England, and was clearly aware of the latest European developments. Mattson reported proudly that "Connoisseurs in the arts have spoken of them in terms of admiration."

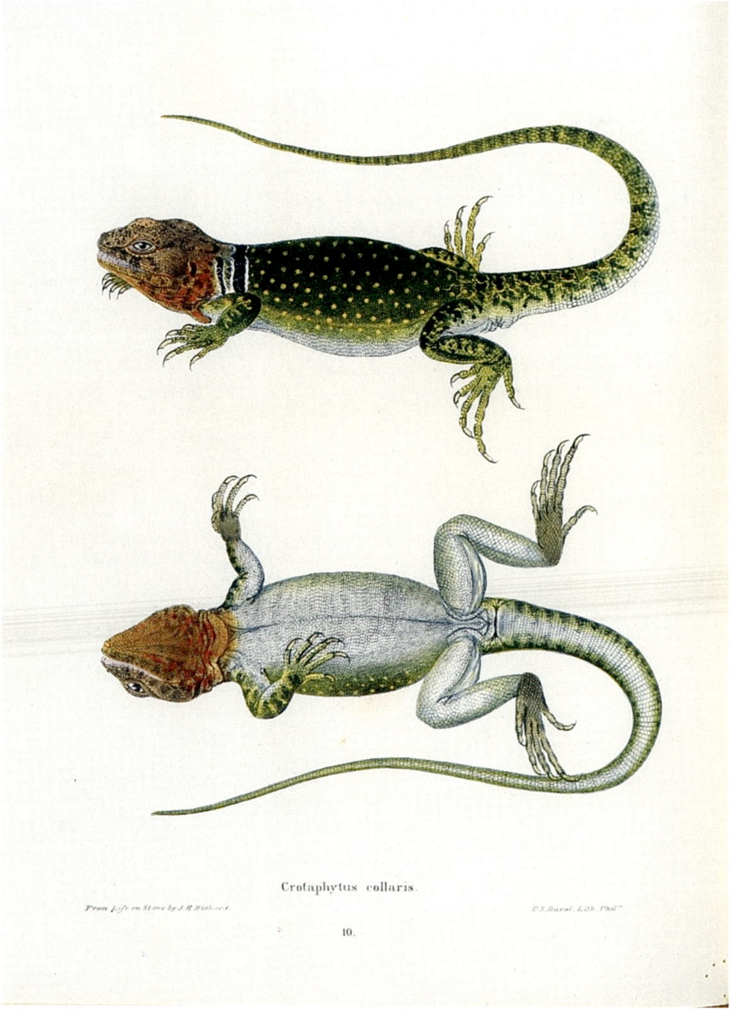

18. John Edward Holbrook: *North American Herpetology; or, a Description of the Reptiles Inhabiting the United States.* Philadelphia: J. Dobson, 1842.

Tinted lithograph with hand coloring

Throughout the era of lithography, Philadelphia remained the most important center for works of natural history involving color plates. The first American work on reptiles was notable for the superb execution and coloring of the plates by Peter S. Duval, whose firm was for decades the leading lithographer and color printer in Philadelphia. Duval executed the plates for both the first edition, issued in 1836–1838, and this second edition of 1842, for which the lithographic stones were entirely redrawn.

As were so many other important figures in the history of American color plate books, Duval was an immigrant, arriving from France in 1831. Many of his workmen were also recruited from Europe, bringing with them knowledge of new technology. Duval, more than any other Philadelphia printer, was involved in plates for book illustration, and he had a well deserved reputation for technical innovation. In this book he included what he called "lithotints," plates with several tones of printed color which were then finished by hand, the originals having been executed directly on stone by J. H. Richard.

19. John Fisk Allen: *Victoria Regia; or the Great Water Lily of America.* Boston. 1854.

Chromolithograph

One of the most striking of American botanical books, this is also among the most successful examples of early chromolithography. William Sharp, the lithographer, had honed his skills since his early and somewhat primitive effort in Mattson's book twelve years before. In the large water lily plates of *Victoria Regia*, Sharp printed colors with a delicacy of execution and technical brilliance never before achieved in the United States. The design of the book and the plates closely followed the earlier English work on the giant water lily by Walter Fitch, issued in 1851.

18. Holbrook, *North American Herpetology. . . .* Tinted lithograph with hand coloring.

20. Charles M. Hovey: *The Fruits of America, Containing Richly Colored Figures, and Full Descriptions of the Choicest Varieties Cultivated in the United States. . . .* New York & Boston: Little, Brown, 1852–1856.

Chromolithograph

Hovey's work on American fruits was the most lavish treatment of the subject prior to the Civil War. The book was sponsored by the Massachusetts Horticultural Society, who turned to William Sharp to produce the beautiful series of chromolithographs which illustrate the work. It was issued in parts, beginning in 1847, and thus can claim to be the first major publication illustrated with chromolithographs. The regular issue, small quarto in size, is exhibited open. Also shown is a copy in original wrappers of the folio large paper issue, of which only eighteen copies were produced. The plates in the large paper version are mounted on stiff card.

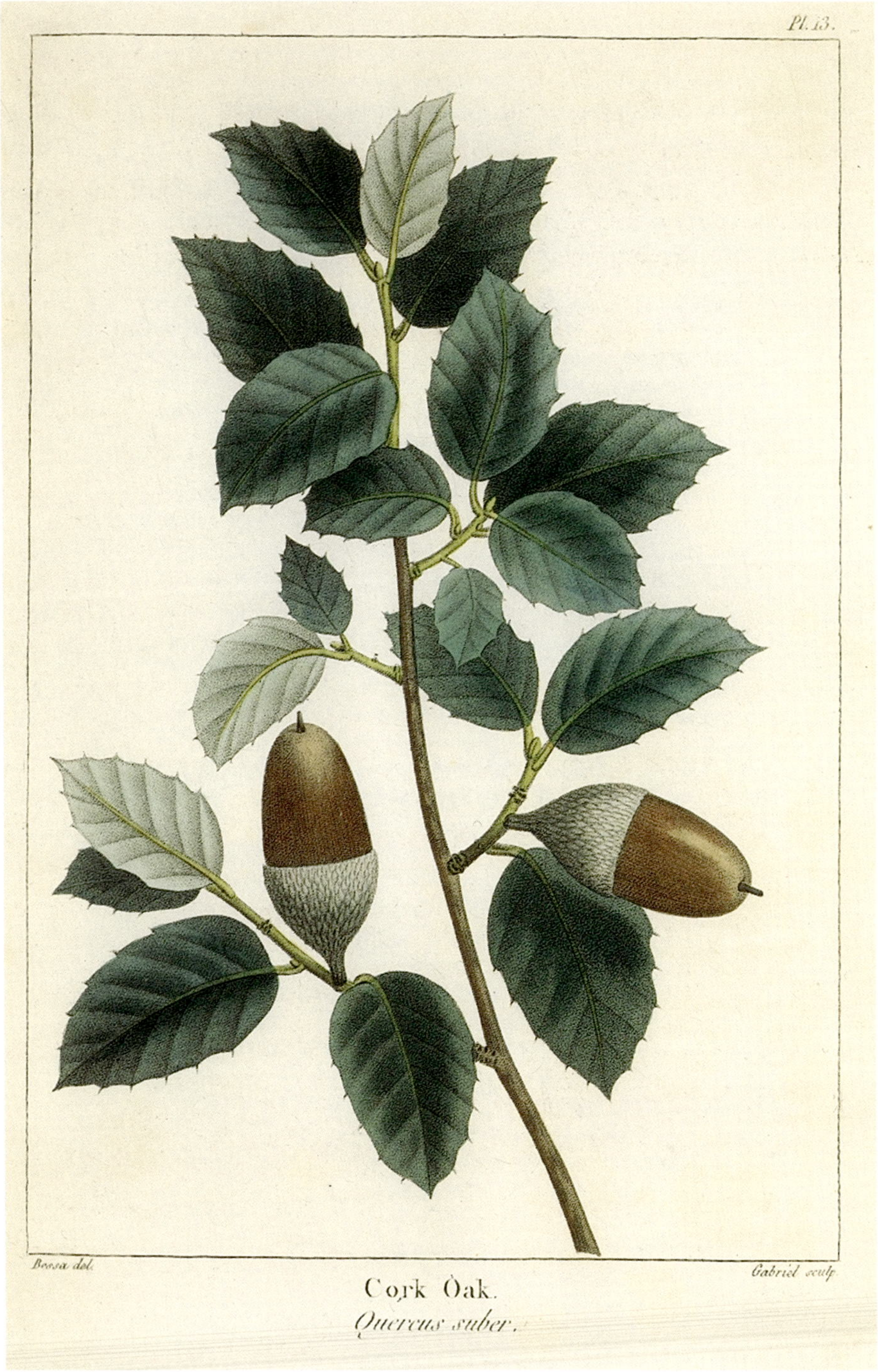

21. Michaux,
The North American Sylva....
Hand-colored stipple engraving.

21. François Andre Michaux: *The North American Sylva; or a Description of the Forest Trees of the United States, Canada, and Nova Scotia....* [with]: Thomas Nuttall: *The North American Sylva...Not Described in the Work of...Michaux.* Philadelphia: Robert P. Smith, 1850–1851.

Michaux: Hand-colored stipple engraving

Few American color plate books had such lasting popularity as this classic work on American trees, or as tangled a publication history. All of the copper plates were made in Paris by the famed French engravers, Redouté and Bessa. They were first published there in 1810–1813, then reprinted in English in 1817–1819, with a false Philadelphia imprint. The plates were purchased by the American naturalist, William Maclure, who took them to New Harmony, Indiana, and produced the first American edition in 1841. He in turn left them to Dr. Samuel G. Morton of Philadelphia, where they were first printed in 1850. As many as ten subsequent editions were issued through 1871, still using the original, but reworked, copper plates.

Nuttall: Hand-colored lithograph

Thomas Nuttall travelled extensively in the South, Midwest, and West between 1815 and 1835. One of his goals was to gather materials to supplement Michaux's work. His book on American trees not covered in Michaux was first issued 1842–1849. This is the second edition, the first uniformly published with Michaux. Nuttall chose lithography as the most practical medium for his plates, which were prepared by the firm of Sinclair in Philadelphia. In 1856 a fire destroyed the premises of the publisher of the joint edition. The Michaux copper plates were saved, but the Nuttall stones were evidently lost, and the later joint editions used new stones.

22. Amos Binney: *The Terrestrial Air-Breathing Mollusks of the United States, and the Adjacent Territories of North America.* Boston: Little, Brown, 1851–1857.

Hand-colored copper plate engraving

Binney, the scion of a wealthy Boston family, was an accomplished amateur naturalist with a particular interest in shells. After his death in 1847, his family subsidized the continuation of his projected book, the plate volume of which did not appear until 1857. Some of the plates had been engraved as early as 1843, by the ubiquitous Alexander Lawson, "who fully understood the views of the author." When Lawson died, the editors felt constrained to go to Paris to find an engraver, since there were no American craftsmen whose work satisfied them. Shown here is a special copy made up for Amos Binney, son of the author, with an uncolored proof facing a finished plate.

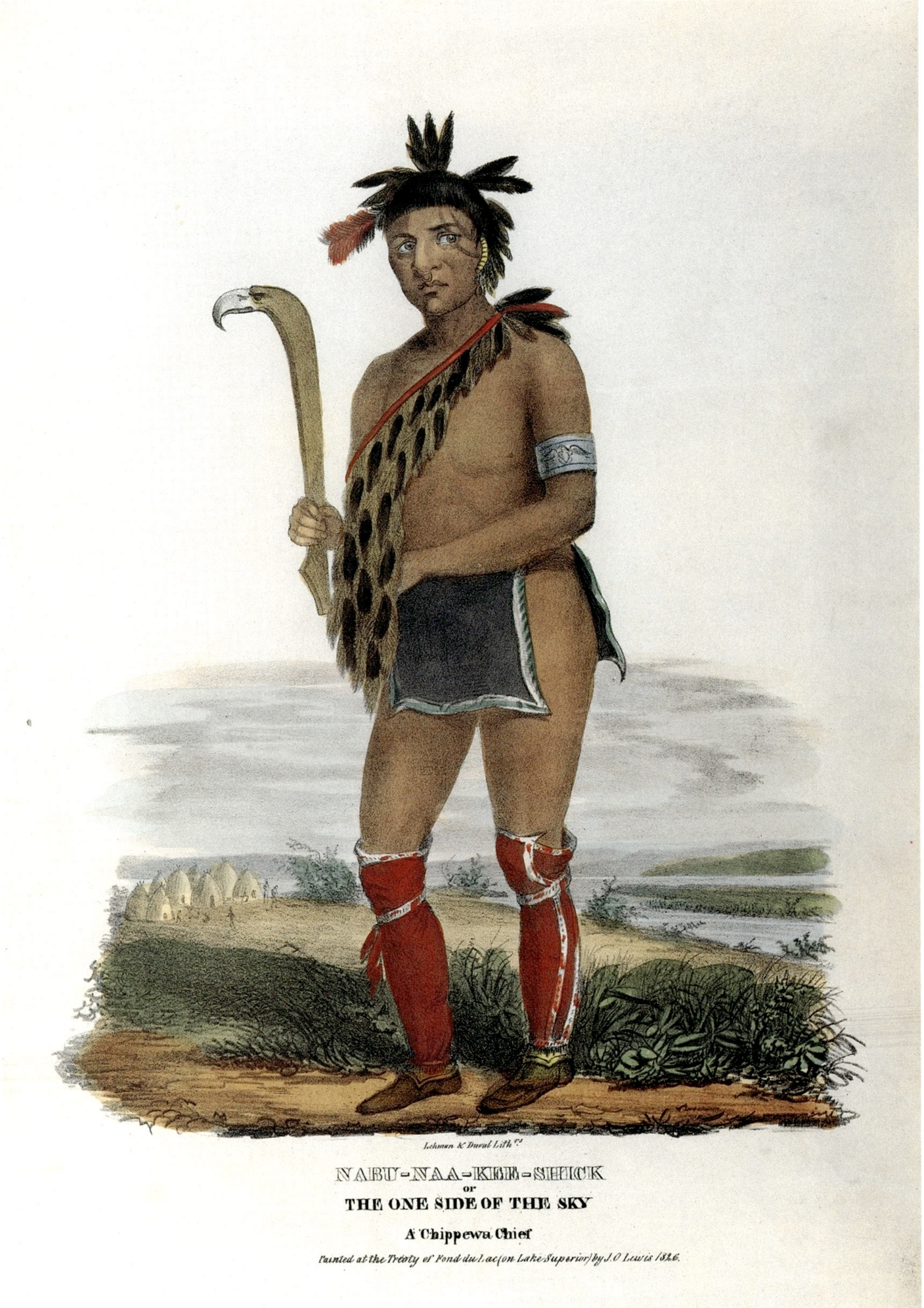

23. Lewis, *The Aboriginal Portfolio.*
Hand-colored lithograph.

CASE 3: Native Americans 1835–1894

Color plate books depicting Native Americans found an audience both in the United States and abroad. The first such publications were two major collections of portraits with biographies, those of James O. Lewis, and McKenney and Hall. The latter, privately published but based on work sponsored by the federal government, remained a perennial favorite, appearing in various editions into the 1880s. Although some early artists, such as George Catlin and Alfred Jacob Miller, based their work on independent travel beyond the United States frontier, most of the color plate work in the field either appeared in official government survey reports, or in private publications by Army officers and government officials, based on their experiences in public service.

23. James Otto Lewis: *The Aboriginal Portfolio.* Philadelphia: [Published by the author], 1835–1836.

Hand-colored lithograph

This was the first attempt made in the United States at a large scale work devoted to the American Indian. Lewis conceived the idea of a folio series of Indian portraits while accompanying Gov. Lewis Cass of Michigan on a tour of the Great Lakes in 1825–1827. He was not able to begin publication until 1835, when the work was advertised as ten parts, each with eight plates, issued in wrappers. The lithographers, George Lehman and Peter S. Duval, did a credible job, but could not overcome the miserable execution of poor Lewis. Subscribers dropped away, and the last two parts are famously rare as a result. The supplement promised in a broadside advertisement never appeared. Nonetheless, it is a pioneering work among such publications.

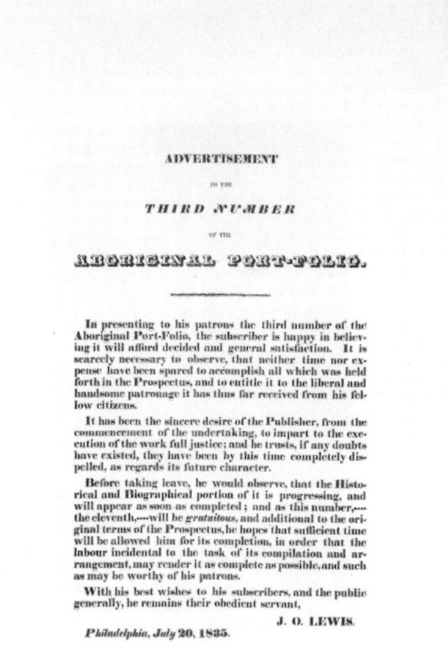

ADVERTISEMENT

TO THE

THIRD NUMBER

OF THE

ABORIGINAL PORT-FOLIO.

In presenting to his patrons the third number of the Aboriginal Port-Folio, the subscriber is happy in believing it will afford decided and general satisfaction. It is scarcely necessary to observe, that neither time nor expense have been spared to accomplish all which was held forth in the Prospectus, and to entitle it to the liberal and handsome patronage it has thus far received from his fellow citizens.

It has been the sincere desire of the Publisher, from the commencement of the undertaking, to impart to the execution of the work full justice; and he trusts, if any doubts have existed, they have been by this time completely dispelled, as regards its future character.

Before taking leave, he would observe, that the Historical and Biographical portion of it is progressing, and will appear as soon as completed; and as this number,—the eleventh,—will be *gratuitous*, and additional to the original terms of the Prospectus, he hopes that sufficient time will be allowed him for its completion, in order that the labour incidental to the task of its compilation and arrangement, may render it as complete as possible, and such as may be worthy of his patrons.

With his best wishes to his subscribers, and the public generally, he remains their obedient servant,

J. O. LEWIS.

Philadelphia, July 20, 1835.

23. Lewis, *The Aboriginal Portfolio.* Prospectus.

24. Thomas L. McKenney and James Hall: *History of the Indian Tribes of North America, with Biographical Sketches and Anecdotes of the Principal Chiefs....* Philadelphia: [Various publishers, including Biddle, Greenough, Rice, and Clark], 1836–1844.

Hand-colored lithograph

With 120 folio plates in three volumes, this was the grandest color plate book issued in the United States up to the time of its publication, and one of the most important of the century. Its long and checkered publication history spanned twelve years and involved multiple lithographers (mainly Peter S. Duval and James T. Bowen) and publishers, but the final product is one of the most distinctive and important books in Americana. Almost all the plates are portraits of individual Native Americans, the majority painted from life by Charles Bird King (who also reworked the less skillful portraits of James Otto Lewis). The complicated circumstances of its production have left a bibliographical stew of issues and issue points that are yet to be satisfactorily resolved.

25. George Catlin: *Catlin's North American Indian Portfolio. Hunting Scenes and Amusements of the Rocky Mountains and Prairies of America.* New York: James Ackerman, 1845.

Hand-colored lithograph

The second great work on American Indians issued in the 1840s was *Catlin's North American Indian Portfolio*. Originally published in London in 1844, this New York 1845 edition was pirated from the English original, evidently without Catlin's knowledge or consent. Not only did the publisher and lithographer, James Ackerman, undersell the author's own edition; he had the cheek to write a preface which criticized Catlin for not publishing the work in the United States, followed by a manifesto proclaiming the ability of American craftsmen to equal the quality of Old World productions. The portfolio was available tinted, colored on paper, or colored mounted on card.

26. George Catlin: [*Catlin's North American Indian Portfolio*...]. New York: Currier & Ives, [ca. 1865].

Hand-colored lithograph

The work of James Ackerman, the cheerful pirate of Catlin's work, appeared in a variety of publications until 1859, when he presumably went out of business. His stock and lithographic stones were evidently dispersed in a way which illustrates how easily material could skip from one publisher to another, especially in the New York printing district. In 1865 the Ackerman Catlin stones reappeared in the hands of Currier & Ives, who altered the captions and credit lines, but left the stones otherwise untouched. Over the next year Currier & Ives published twenty-four individual plates for fifty cents each. The stone for the twenty-fifth plate was presumably lost or broken between 1845 and 1865.

27. Henry Trumbull: *History of the Discovery of America, of the Landing of our Forefathers, at Plymouth, and of their Most Remarkable Engagements with the Indians, in New-England.* Boston: Published by George Clark, 1840.

Hand-colored woodcut

Concurrent with the elegant folios of Catlin, and McKenney and Hall, a more popular type of book used cheap colored woodcuts to convey the horrors of Indian warfare. Among the most frequently reprinted was this history, written when the author was seventeen. The gaudy frontispiece illustrates the Battle of the Thames in the War of 1812. Later editions supplied new woodcuts to be more up to date, featuring Seminole War conflicts. Numerous popular histories were produced in the 1840s and 1850s, utilizing hastily applied blotchy color on woodcuts, evidently with the theory that any color was better than none.

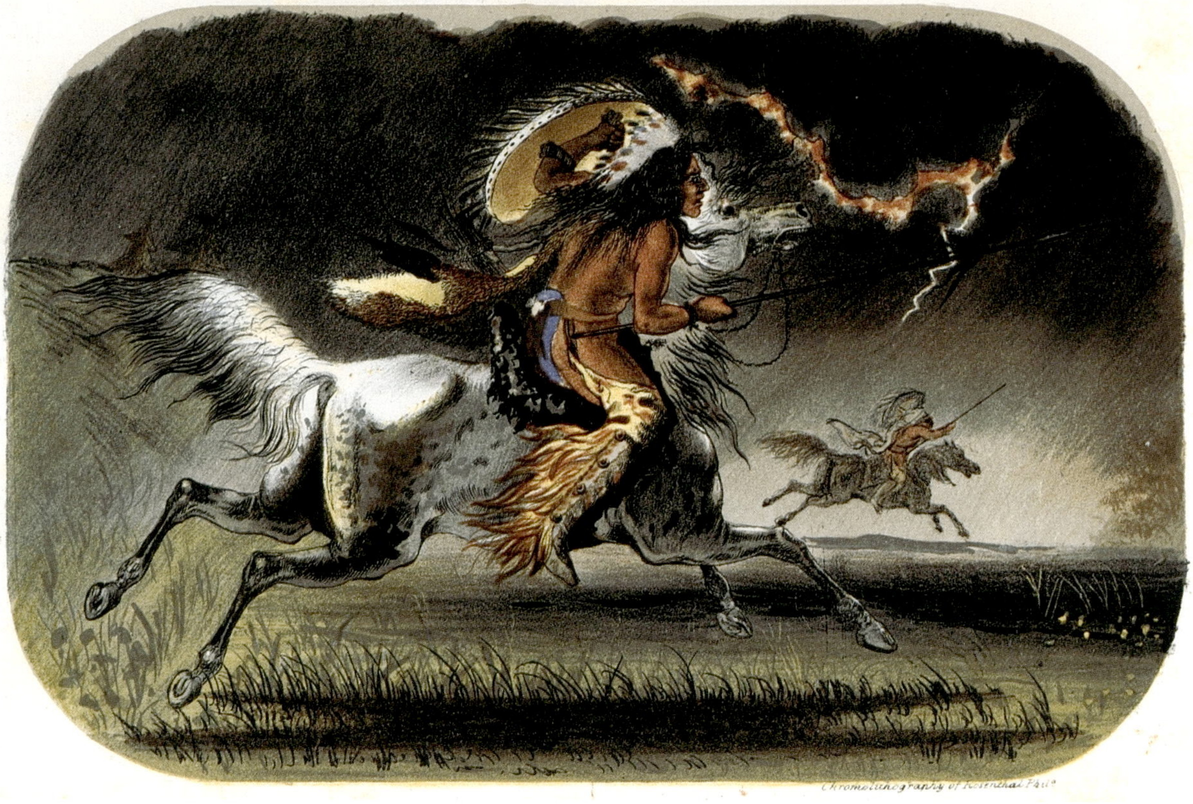

28. Webber,
Wild Scenes and Song-Birds.
Chromolithograph.

28. Charles W. Webber: *Wild Scenes and Song-Birds.* New York: George P. Putnam, 1854.

Chromolithograph

Another artist who lived among Native Americans and painted them beyond the bounds of civilization was Alfred Jacob Miller, a young painter who went to Wyoming in 1837 with the British soldier and sportsman, Sir William Drummond Stewart. After the publication of his edition of Catlin, James Ackerman advertised that he was planning a folio work with fifty plates based on Miller's work. Sadly, this never came to pass, and the only publication Miller achieved, a pale reflection of what might have been, were five plates in this hodgepodge volume of hunting stories and natural history lore. The plates were executed by one of the first chromolithographers in Philadelphia, Louis Rosenthal.

29. James H. Simpson: *Journal of a Military Reconnaissance, from Santa Fe, New Mexico, to the Navajo Country. . . .* Philadelphia: Lippincott, Grambo, 1852.

Chromolithograph

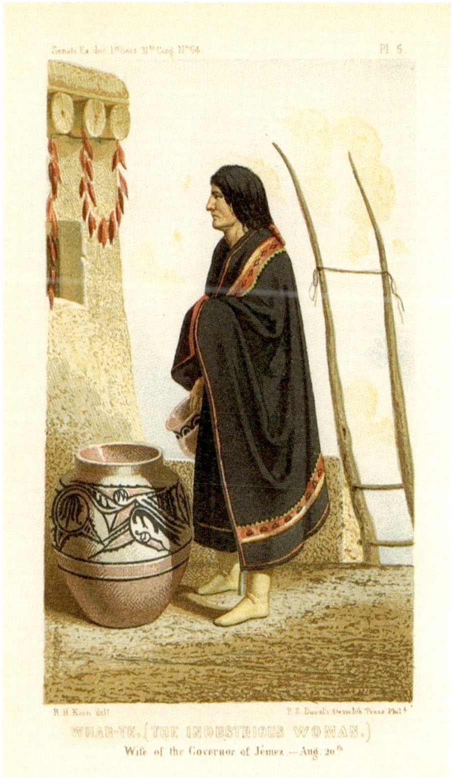

29. Simpson, *Journal of a Military Reconnaissance. . . .* Chromolithograph.

Lieutenant Simpson led an expedition northwest from Santa Fe in 1849, accompanied by the artist, Richard Kern. His report published some of the earliest views of the Pueblos, a topic of consuming interest for American artists ever since. This report also mixed chromolithographs, hand-colored lithographs, and uncolored lithographs, all from the shop of Peter S. Duval. It was among the earliest of government-sponsored explorations in the American West to be extensively illustrated with color plates.

30. John S. Hart, ed.: *The Iris. An Illuminated Souvenir for 1852.* Philadelphia: Lippincott, Grambo, 1852.

Chromolithograph

Produced in full Victorian splendor, this gift book was mainly a vehicle for the romantic fictions of Indian life in Minnesota by Mary Eastman and accompanying illustrations by her soldier-painter husband, Capt. Seth Eastman. The editor proudly boasted that the lithographer, Peter S. Duval, used ten separate stones to create the chromolithographs, overprinting some colors to create varied effects. The result shows the difficulty even the best craftsmen still had in controlling so many colors; or perhaps, as Daniel McGrath commented, "Duval selected for the printing colors guaranteed to appeal to the insensate."

31. William H. Emory: *Report on the United States and Mexican Boundary Survey, Made under the Direction of the Secretary of the Interior. . . .* Washington: Cornelius Wendell, Printer, 1857–1859.

Chromolithograph

Emory's report on surveying the new boundary with Mexico after the Mexican War demonstrates the broad range of mediums available by the 1850s to convey graphic information. There are three separate mediums of color used. The plates depicting Native Americans are chromolithographs, while the twenty-five ornithology plates are hand-colored lithographs, and other natural history plates utilize hand-colored steel engravings. Uncolored illustrations are woodcuts, lithographs, and steel engravings. Emory provided the first visual images of the tribes of Arizona.

32. Richard I. Dodge: *Our Wild Indians: Thirty-three Years' Personal Experience among the Red Men of the Great West. . . .* Hartford: A. D. Worthington and Co., 1883.

Chromolithograph

Dodge spent all of his army career, excepting the Civil War, on the western frontier. By the time he wrote this book, published by a Hartford subscription house, any menace posed by the western tribes was over. Perhaps significantly, the elaborate chromolithographs illustrating the work are devoted entirely to artifacts which had already passed into the realm of legend and collectibility: a dress decorated with elk teeth is described in the caption as having a value of $200. These handsome chromolithographic plates would have been prominently shown in the salesman's dummies issued by the subscription houses, as an inducement to purchase.

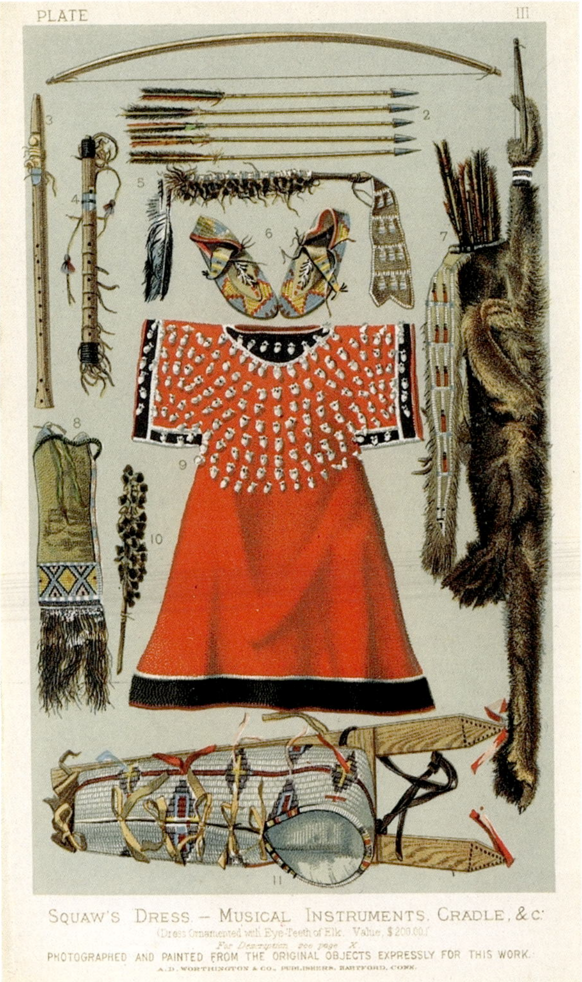

33. Donaldson,
Reports on Indians Taxed and Not Taxed....
Chromolithograph.

ELEVENTH CENSUS OF THE UNITED STATES.
ROBERT P. PORTER, SUPERINTENDENT.

INDIANS.

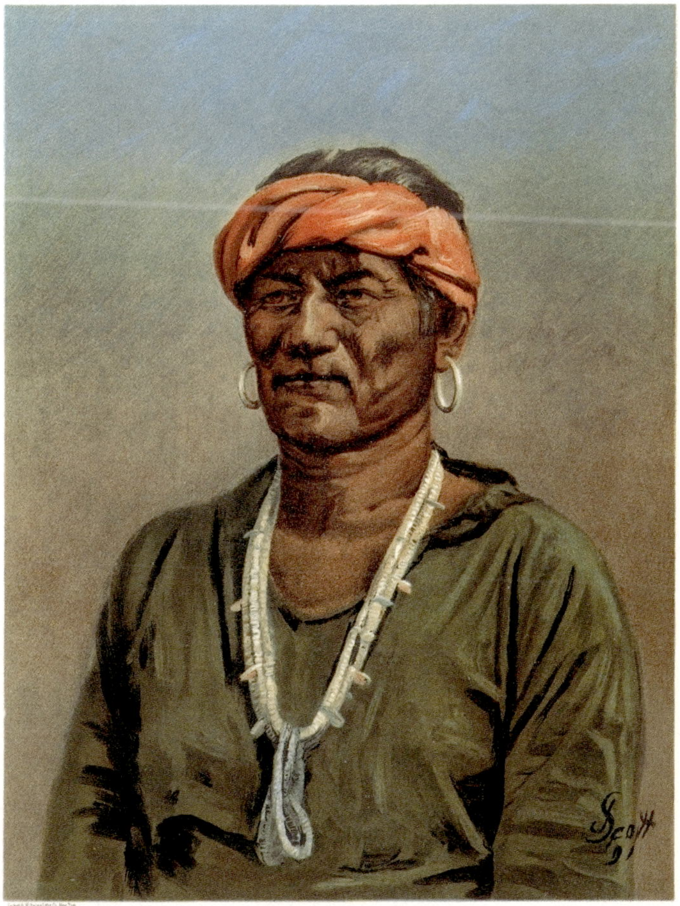

MANULETO.
CHIEF OF THE NAVAJOS.—ARIZONA, 1891.

32. Dodge,
Our Wild Indians....
Chromolithograph.

33. Thomas C. Donaldson, ed.: *Reports on Indians Taxed and Not Taxed....* Washington: Government Printing Office, 1894.

Chromolithograph

The Eleventh Census in 1890 undertook the first systematic effort by the U.S. government to record the Native Americans within its borders. The elaborate report continued a tradition already begun by the annual reports of the Bureau of American Ethnology in the 1880s, providing a range of illustrations including chromolithographs. The artist, Julian Scott, was commissioned to produce a series of portraits of notable individuals, printed by the New York firm of Sackett & Wilhelms.

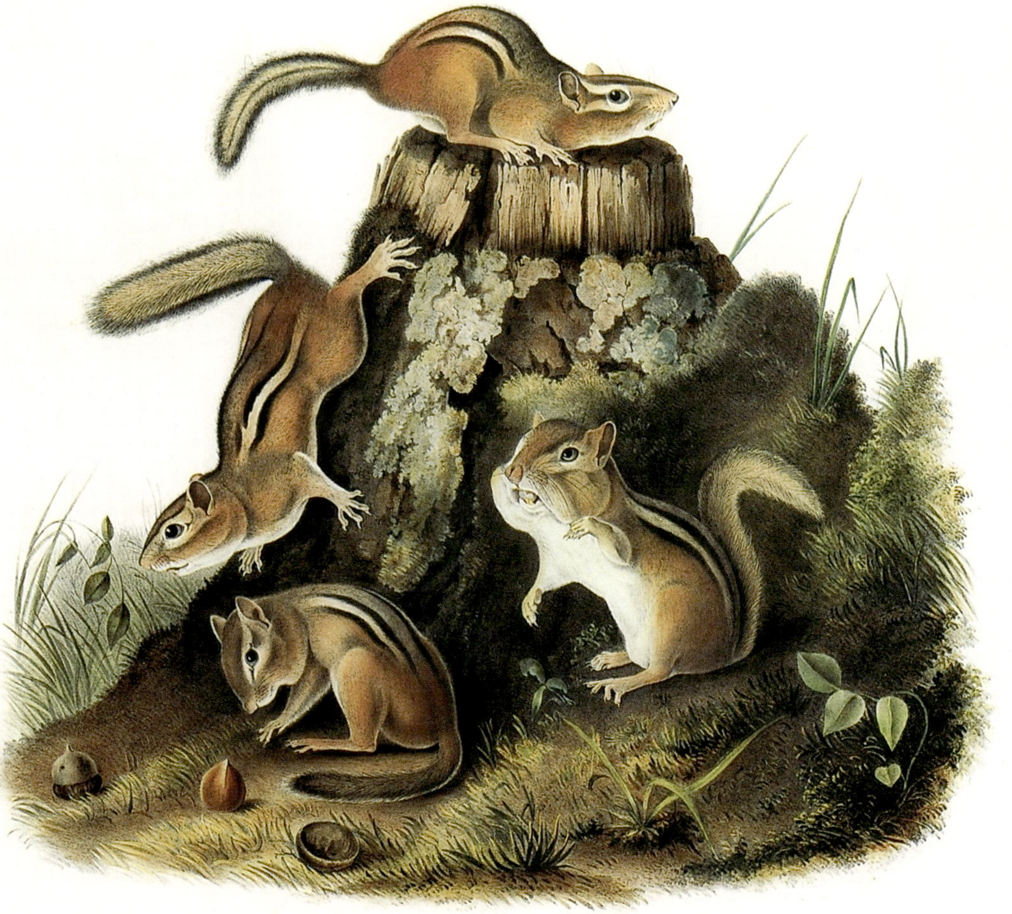

37. Audubon,
[*Proof Plate for the Folio Edition of the* Quadrupeds].
Hand-colored lithograph.

CASE 4: The Audubons 1840–1870

The publishing enterprises of John James Audubon and his sons, Victor and John Woodhouse, encompass a range of superlatives in 19th-century American color plate books. Together they produced what was probably the greatest commercial success of the genre, the octavo edition of *The Birds of America.* They went on to the largest commercially viable project of the century, the folio and octavo editions of *The Quadrupeds of North America.* Finally, after the death of his father and brother, J. W. Audubon undertook a reprinting *The Birds of America* in its original elephant folio size. Although only one-third of the project was completed, the so-called Bien Audubon (after the printer, Julius Bien) is the largest single color plate book of the century. The Audubons and their works are at the heart of the story of the color plate book in America.

34. John James Audubon: *The Birds of America, from Drawings Made in the United States and Their Territories.* New York & Philadelphia: J. J. Audubon and J. B. Chevalier, 1840–44.

Hand-colored lithograph

The octavo edition of Audubon's *Birds* was probably the greatest commercial success of any color plate book issued in 19th-century America. While Audubon had become internationally famous in the course of producing the double elephant folio edition of the *Birds* in London between 1826 and 1839, it was this octavo version, issued at $100, which achieved widespread circulation and brought the work into the homes of many well-to-do Americans. Originally issued in one hundred parts, the set was published over a five-year period and was complete in seven volumes. All of the lithographs were made by the firm of J. T. Bowen in Philadelphia.

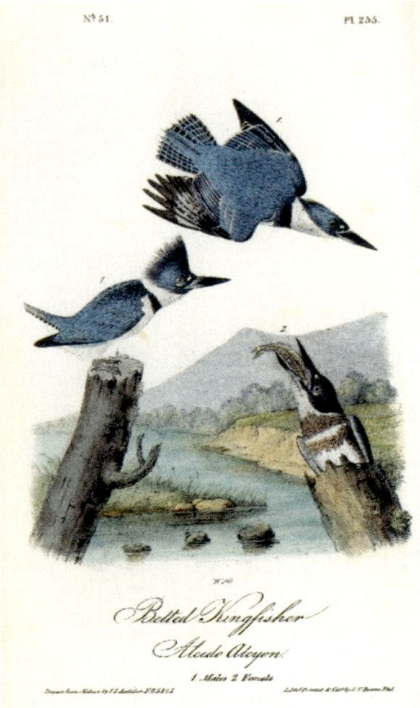

34. Audubon,
The Birds of America....
Hand-colored lithograph.

35. John James Audubon: *The Birds of America....* New York: Roe, Lockwood, 1861.

Tinted lithograph with hand coloring

There were eight subsequent editions of the octavo *Birds*, the last appearing in 1889. All of these are distinguished by having several tint stones printed on most of the plates prior to the application of hand coloring. This reduced the amount of hand coloring applied to each plate. The earlier reprint editions were as carefully executed as the original, but after the copyright of the work passed into the hands of Roe, Lockwood in New York, production standards slipped. The quality of color in this 1861 edition does not compare to that of 1840.

36. John James Audubon and John Bachman: *The Viviparous Quadrupeds of North America.* New York: J. J. Audubon, 1845–1848.

Hand-colored lithograph

By 1843 the Audubon family business was a well oiled machine, involving John James, his two sons, Victor and John Woodhouse, and various in-laws and friends. The octavo *Birds* was still in production when J. T. Bowen began to produce the plates for the elephant folio edition of the *Quadrupeds*, the largest successful color plate book project of 19th-century America. It took the family five years to publish 150 plates in thirty parts. The massive project was a commercial success, thanks to the close management of Victor. There were about three hundred subscribers.

37. John James Audubon: [*Proof Plate for the Folio Edition of the* Quadrupeds]. Philadelphia: J. T. Bowen, 1843.

Hand-colored lithograph

The first proofs of the folio edition of the *Quadrupeds* were struck in the summer of 1843, when John James Audubon left on his last expedition, a journey up the Missouri River to see the Far West. Although little of scientific value was achieved, the old man was lionized by the fur traders and army officers he met along the way and enjoyed himself greatly. He took with him colored proof plates, before letters, of the first fifteen plates of the new book, dispensing them as gifts to his new friends. This plate of the "American Chipmunk" was given to a young Army lieutenant, James Henry Carleton, who took Audubon buffalo hunting near Fort Union.

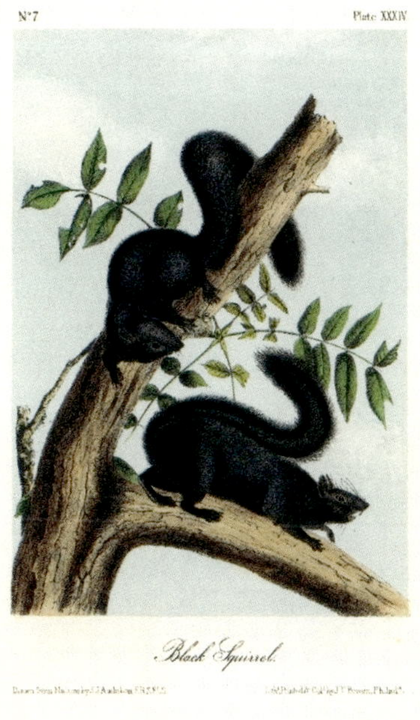

38. Audubon, *The Quadrupeds of North America.* Hand-colored lithograph.

38. John James Audubon and John Bachman: *The Quadrupeds of North America.* New York: Published by V. G. Audubon, 1849–1854.

Hand-colored lithograph

As with the octavo edition of the *Birds*, the octavo *Quadrupeds* appealed to a larger audience and sold far more copies than the folio edition. The Audubon family business of art and natural history rolled on, beginning production of the octavo edition with J. T. Bowen as soon as the folio plates were finished. It appeared in thirty-one parts between 1849 and 1854. During this time Bowen was also kept busy reprinting plates needed to complete sets of the octavo *Birds*, while the brothers took turns canvassing the country for subscriptions.

39. John James Audubon: *The Quadrupeds of North America.* New York: George R. Lockwood, [1871].

Uncolored lithograph

The octavo *Quadrupeds*, almost as popular as the octavo *Birds*, also went through a number of editions. The copyrights on all of the octavo editions seem to have passed into the control of the firm of Roe, Lockwood in the course of the Audubon family bankruptcy in 1862. This later edition, with the plates uncolored, shows what a typical plate would have looked like before hand coloring was applied.

40. John James Audubon: *The Birds of America. From Drawings Made in the United States and Their Territories.* New York: Roe, Lockwood & Son, 1861.

Chromolithograph finished with hand coloring

In 1858 John Woodhouse Audubon undertook the task of reprinting, in chromolithography, *The Birds of America* on the same scale as the original double elephant folio. The German immigrant lithographer, Julius Bien, was hired to print the work. Although only one-third completed when the project collapsed in 1861, the Bien Audubon is the largest and most ambitious color plate book undertaken in 19th-century America, rivaled only by the folio *Quadrupeds.* The onset of the Civil War caused many subscribers to withdraw, and precipitated the bankruptcy of the Audubon family and the death of J. W. Audubon from overwork. The plates were taken over by the firm of Roe, Lockwood, who also seem to have obtained the copyright of the other Audubon books at this point.

Bien had great difficulty controlling tones and colors in the large plates, and some seem flat and lack fine detail. It is probable that J. W. Audubon and Bien always intended that plates would be hand finished with color and gum arabic, as in the copy exhibited, creating a wholly different impression on the viewer. When the Audubon family and Bien lost control of the project and the plates passed into the control of Roe, Lockwood, this was not done, since sets and plates were then marketed in a remainder fashion. The few finished copies show what might have been.

41. John Woodhouse Audubon: *Illustrated Notes of an Expedition through Mexico and California....* New York: Published by J. W. Audubon, 1852.

Hand-colored lithograph

In 1849 John Woodhouse Audubon joined the gold rush, travelling to California across Texas and northern Mexico. On his return, he planned an ambitious plate book of forty plates in ten parts, illustrating scenes from his trip and in the mines. Despite the tremendous national interest in the gold rush, he was unable to generate enough subscriptions to justify the publication, and so packaged the whole letterpress text, with the plates of the projected first part, as a complete book. Even the Audubon family's ability to market could not overcome the reluctance of American audiences to pay the cost of large view books.

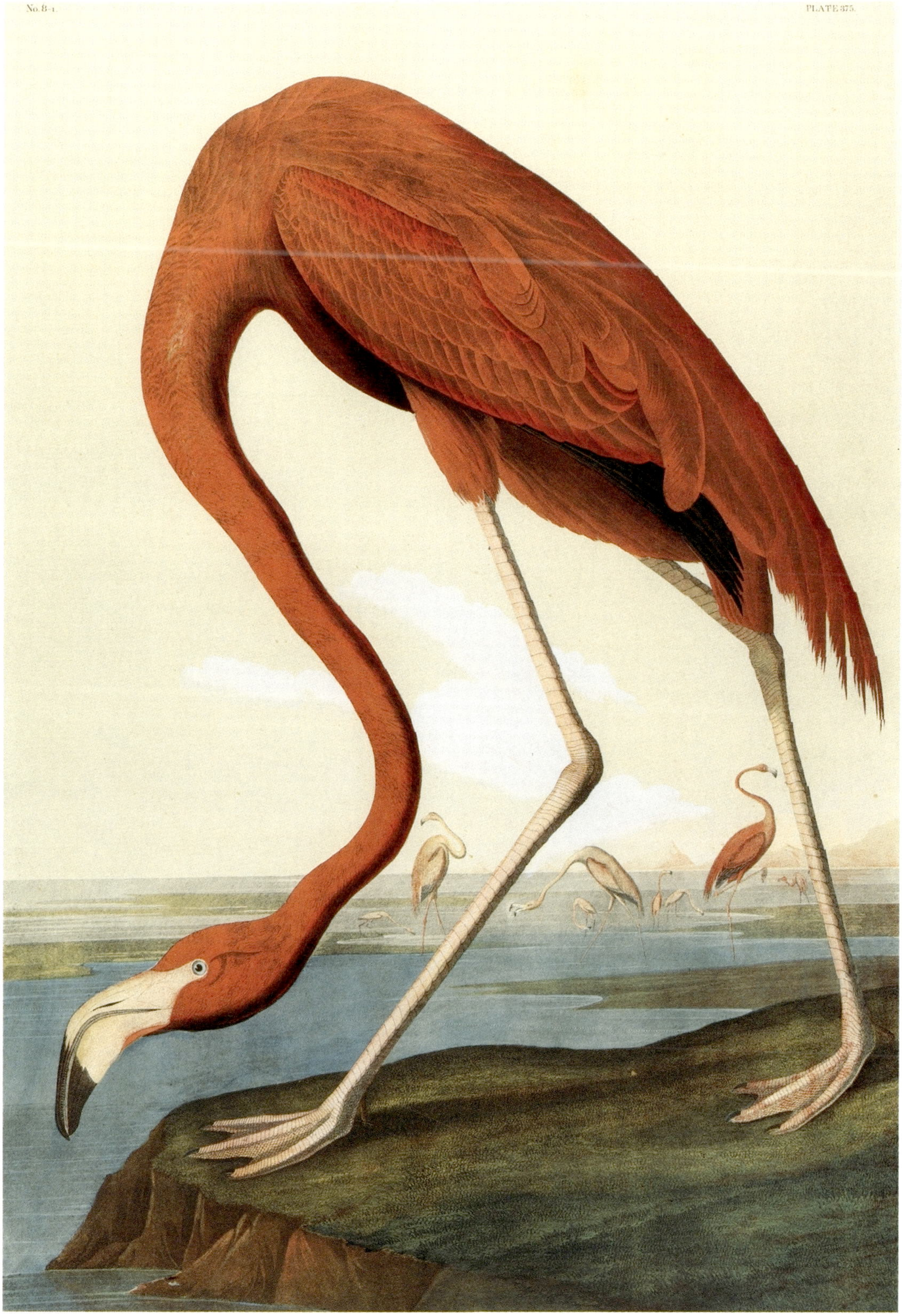

40. Audubon, *The Birds of America.*
Chromolithograph finished with hand coloring.

42. John Cassin: *Illustrations of the Birds of California, Texas, Oregon, British and Russian America. Intended to Contain Descriptions and Figures of All North American Birds Not Given by Former American Authors, and a General Synopsis of North American Ornithology.* Philadelphia: J. B. Lippincott & Co., [1853]–1856.

Hand-colored lithograph

John Cassin, a Philadelphia ornithologist who had travelled extensively in the West, approached the Audubon brothers in the summer of 1851 with a proposal to create a supplement to the octavo *Birds* in three further volumes. With their father dead, Victor and John Woodhouse were in full command of the family enterprises. At first the Audubons were receptive, already planning for the next project to follow the octavo *Quadrupeds*. However, Cassin wanted shared credit on the title page and a free hand in correcting the errors of nomenclature of the elder Audubon, a touchy point with the sons. In the end, Cassin went on his own, although clearly following the Audubon format and also using J. T. Bowen as lithographer.

43. Juan Lembeye: *Aves de la Isla de Cuba.* Havana: Imprenta del Tiempo, 1850.

Hand-colored lithograph

The success and fame of the Audubon publications caused their images to be widely copied and reworked. This is one of the more unusual instances of pirating from *The Birds of America*, in a work about the birds of Cuba published in Havana a few years after the octavo *Birds* came out. The author, who supplied a competent ornithological text, had a Havana lithographer lift the illustrations straight from Audubon.

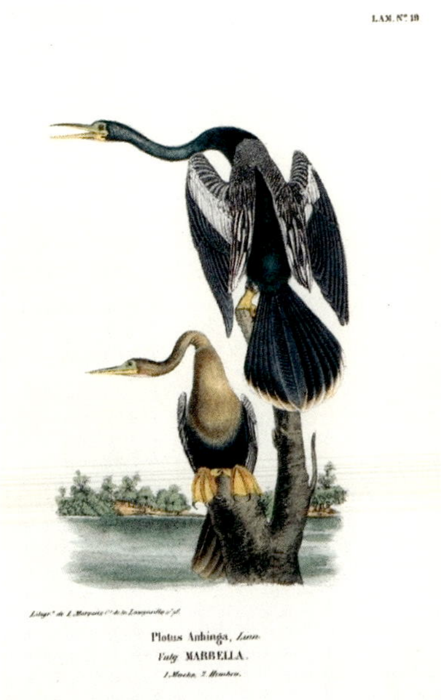

43. Lembeye,
Aves de la Isla de Cuba.
Hand-colored lithograph.

44. Daniel Giraud Elliot: *The New and Heretofore Unfigured Species of the Birds of North America.* New York: Published by the author, 1866–1869.

Hand-colored lithograph

Besides Cassin, the other great ornithologist in the Audubon tradition was Daniel G. Elliot. He, too, sought to add to the species described in *The Birds of*

44. Elliot, *The New . . . Birds of North America.* Hand-colored lithograph.

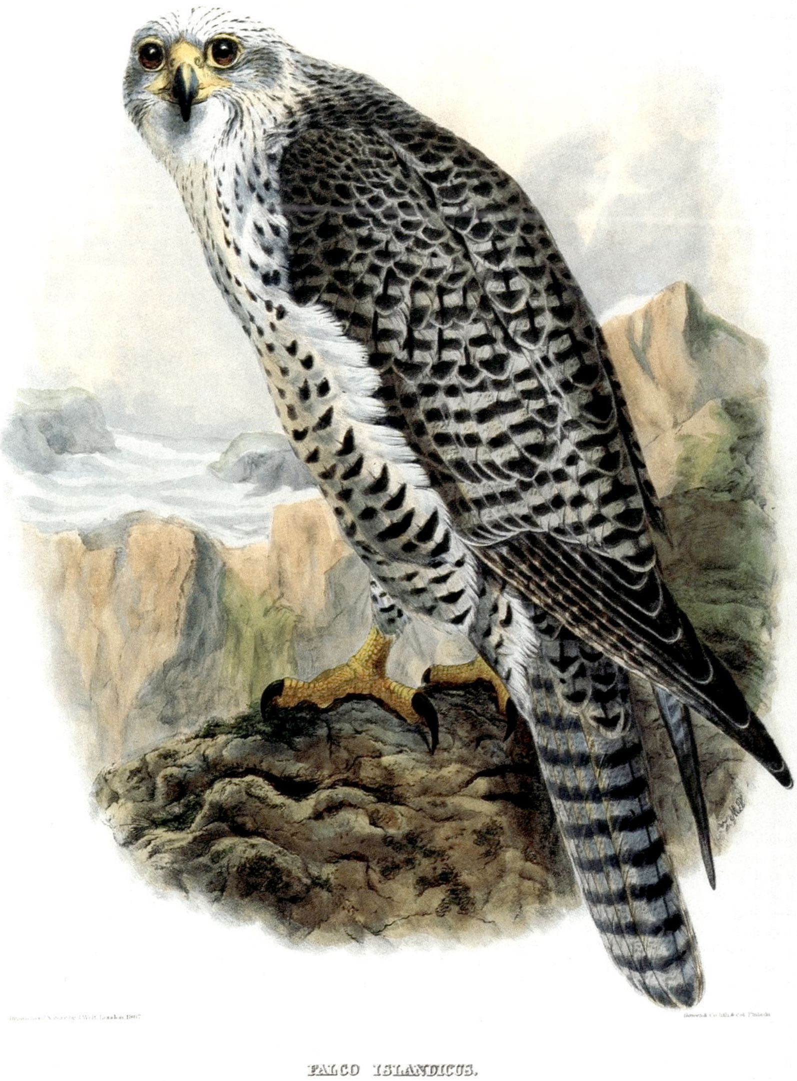

America, as the title of his largest work suggests. By 1869, the Bowen firm was the only shop left in the United States capable of undertaking a work on this scale with hand-colored lithographs, the medium Elliot required. After the demise of J. T. Bowen, his widow married John Cassin and carried on the business. They also produced Elliot's works on American grouse (1865) and antthrushes (1867). The Bowen firm closed after this book completed publication in 1869. Elliot moved to Europe and had the plates for the rest of his books produced in Belgium, although he continued to use a New York imprint.

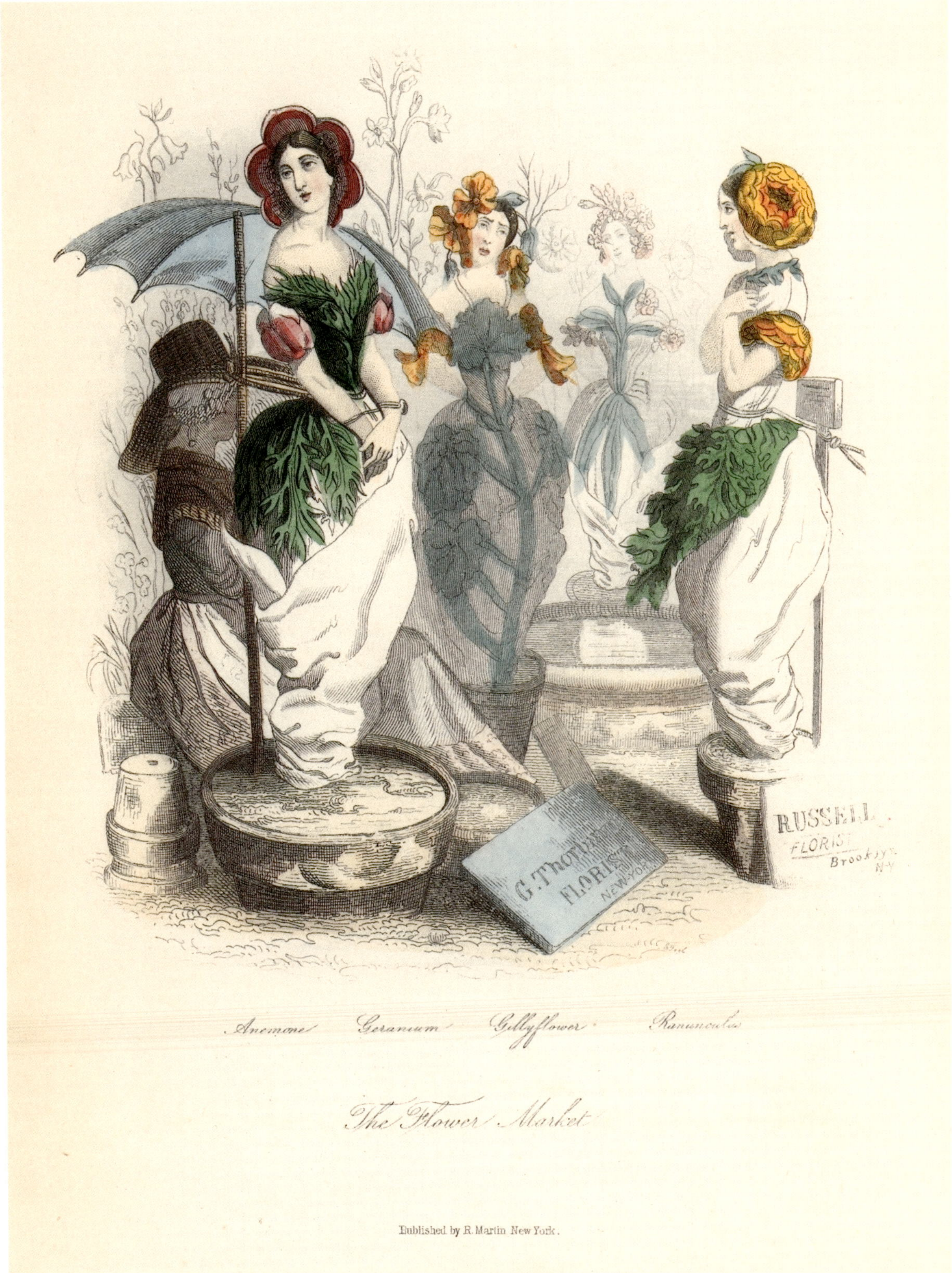

55. Grandville, *The Flowers Personified.*
Hand-colored steel engraving.

CASE 5: Fashion and Sentiment 1813–1885

In the early decades of the 19th century, color plates were so expensive that their appearance, with a few small exceptions, was limited to relatively large and costly works. By the late 1830s, color work was more affordable, and color could be used to enhance a range of of publications more lighthearted in nature. The decades before the Civil War saw a boom in color fashion plates and a craze for illustrated gift books, literary annuals enhanced with color plates, and similar "sentimental" books. The inclusion of color in such books was an enhancement which also acted as a powerful sales tool. They brought color plates from the realm of science, natural history, and the library, into the parlor and everyday life.

45. [Anonymous]: *Mirror of the Graces.* [New York: I. Riley, 1813].

Hand-colored copper plate engraving

This little book is the first American publication with color plates devoted to fashion and etiquette. The extreme modesty of its four duodecimo plates gives a better idea of the real beginnings of color plate books in America than Birch's large and accomplished productions. Color plates were an expensive addition for any publisher to contemplate, and their sparse use in productions such as this were much more the rule than the few grand projects of the first quarter of the century.

46. [Pennsylvania Militia]: *The Soldier's Manual, for the Cavalry, Artillery, Light Infantry, and Infantry. Embellished with Twelve Plates, Representing Different Volunteer Corps, in the First Division Pennsylvania Militia.* Philadelphia: Published by James H. Nesmith, 1824.

Hand-colored copper plate engraving

The first military costume book produced in the United States depicted the uniforms of the Pennsylvania militia. It is a hybrid production, since the text is that of a standard military manual. The plates show off the handsome uniforms of the different state militia units. As with fashion plates, the best military costume plates of the pre-Civil War era appear in periodicals, notably the *United States Military Magazine.*

47. Mrs. A. Walker: *Female Beauty, as Preserved and Improved by Regimen, Cleanliness and Dress; and Especially by the Adaptation, Colour and Arrangement of Dress, as Variously Influencing the Forms, Complexion, and Expression of each Individual, and Rendering Cosmetic Impositions Unnecessary.* New York: Scofield and Voorhies, [1840?].

Hand-colored lithograph

47. Walker, *Female Beauty...*
Hand-colored lithograph.

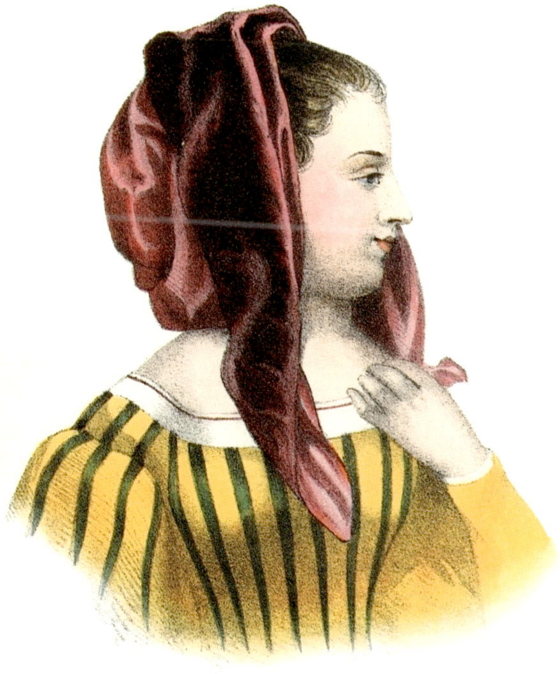

American publishers seemed to depend on the English and French to supply ideas of correct taste and the forms in which to express it. This handbook of fashion and behavior uses overlaid color plates, with a cut-out in the upper plate, to show the effects of different colors in clothes with light or dark complexions. Although issued by a New York publisher, the plates were produced by J. T. Bowen in Philadelphia. The title page asserts that the book, pirated from an English publisher, was "Revised and Amended by an American Editor," although it is hard to say how. Americans seemed split between a desire to ape European fashion and chauvinistic pride in their country.

48. [F. Quarre]: *The Artist.* New York: Herald Printing Establishment, 1842–1843.

Color-printed aquatint; color-printed aquatint with hand coloring

Quarre's fashion periodical, which only survived for twelve issues, exemplifies the experimentation with color printing techniques in book illustration which paralleled the beginnings of chromolithography in the 1840s. The publisher claimed that his plates were "engravings in color...the invention and the means of execution are our own exclusive property...we shall have been the first to trace out a new line, which has not yet been attempted in any other country...."

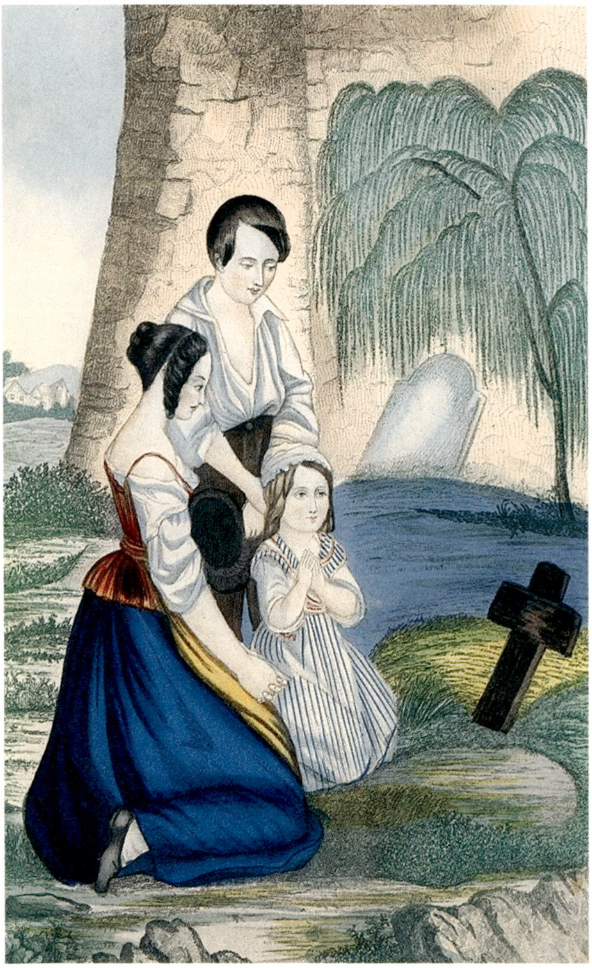

48. [Quarre], *The Artist.* Color-printed aquatint with hand coloring.

Although difficult to determine exactly, the plates appear to be aquatints, some entirely color printed and others partly printed and partly hand-colored. The volume also contains instances of full hand coloring.

49. [Frank Leslie]: *Frank Leslie's Ladies Gazette of Fashion and the Beau Monde.* New York: Frank Leslie, 1855.

Hand-colored steel engraving

Surprisingly few books devoted to fashion were published in 19th-century America. Virtually all of the many costume and fashion plates appeared in periodicals, generally with one colored plate per issue. The most famous of these were *Godey's Ladies Book* and *Peterson's National Ladies' Magazine*, in their heyday during the 1840s and 1850s. The most lavish, however, was Leslie's *Gazette of Fashion*, produced on a larger format and with more accomplished plates than its competitors.

50. M. Augustin Challamel: *The History of Fashion in France or the Dress of Women from the Gallo-Roman Period to the Present Time.* New York: Scribner & Welford, 1882.

Hand-colored copper plate engraving

European fashion remained the touchstone for elegant dress in the United States throughout the century. This book is both an example of the fascination with French couture and the degree to which American color plate work stood in the shadow of European craftsmanship. The plates for this book were printed in Paris and imported, while the rest of the work was produced in New York. Numerous publishers undertook the expense of importing plates throughout the 19th century, presumably finding it cheaper or better than American production – perhaps both.

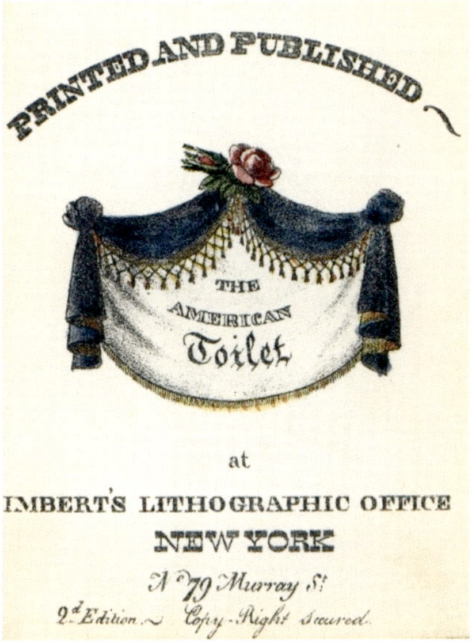

51. [Anonymous], *The American Toilet.* Hand-colored lithograph.

51. [Anonymous]: *The American Toilet.* New York: Imbert's Lithographic Office, [ca. 1827].

Hand-colored lithograph

Small gift books were already popular in England in the 1820s, and the lithographer, Imbert, blatantly pirated a British work to produce his *American Toilet.* In this delicate little work, the illustrations of various cosmetic canisters have hinged flaps of paper which can be raised to see the "true" beautifier. Thus "A Wash to Smooth Away Wrinkles" is revealed to be "laughter," "Genuine Rouge" to be "modesty," and so forth.

52. Elizabeth Washington Gamble Wirt: *Flora's Dictionary . . . Embellished by Mrs. Anna Smith.* Baltimore: Fielding Lucas, Jr., 1837.

Hand-colored lithograph

One of the most popular genres of color plate books in the antebellum period were those devoted to the sentiments associated with flowers. Colored illustrations of flowers were accompanied by a text which guided the reader through the hidden meanings of different blooms, with quotations and poetry appropriate to each. This is a pioneering example of the type, issued by the publisher of many early books with color, Fielding Lucas of Baltimore. Similar works were issued at every level of quality and size, from pocket-sized volumes with crude plates to highly finished folios.

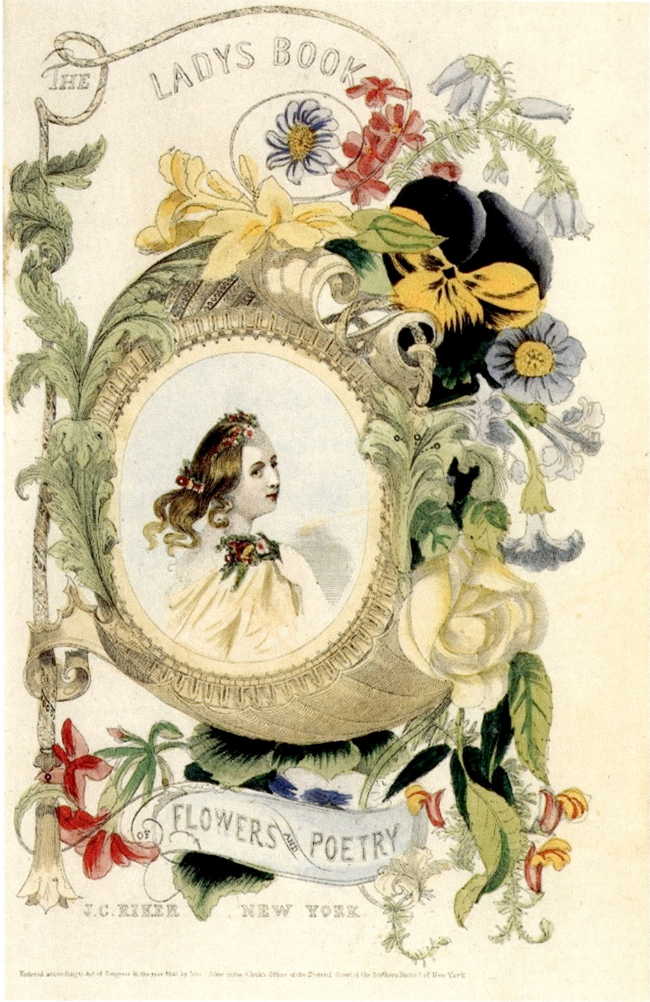

53. Hooper,
The Lady's Book of Flowers and Poetry....
Hand-colored steel engraving.

53. Lucy Hooper: *The Lady's Book of Flowers and Poetry; to which Are Added, a Botanical Introduction, a Complete Floral Dictionary; and a Chapter on Plants in Rooms.* New York: J. C. Riker, 1843.

Hand-colored lithograph; hand-colored steel engraving

Lucy Hooper, a Brooklyn poet who died at a tragically young age, perfected the formula of the gift book with this work, which first appeared in 1842 and went through numerous editions. Tasteful floral color plates were combined with selected poems of early Victorian poets, essays on the meaning of flowers, and a handsome binding. Sentimentality fairly oozed from its covers. The printer of the plates, J. C. Riker, repackaged his work in other forms, such as blank notebooks, with the same floral illustrations bound in. While the plates are lithographs, the elaborate title is a steel engraving.

54. Alfred A. Phillips, ed.: *The Forget-Me-Not: a Gift for 1846.* New York: Nafis & Cornish, 1846.

Chromolithograph, hand-colored lithograph

Gift books appeared in myriad forms in the decades preceding the Civil War, reaching the height of their appeal about 1850. This small volume is an example of the more modest end of the genre. The plates were crudely produced in chromolithography, occasionally heightened with hand-applied color. Even a few color plates added sparkle.

55. F. L. Grandville: *The Flowers Personified: Being a Translation of Grandville's "Les Fleurs Animees."* New York: Published by R. Martin, 1847–1849.

Hand-colored steel engraving

Grandville's work was originally published in Paris, and its European editions achieved wide circulation. The steel plates for this American edition were cut, with some changes from the Paris original, in New York. The publisher could not resist adding the names of several New York florists to the plate of "The Flower Market." The early Victorian notions of the sentiments of flowers reach a bizarre climax in this book. Not only are the flowers at market depicted as bound maidens, but other plates show virginal flower maids running shrieking from anthropomorphized shears, and a Hemlock maiden administering a fatal draught to a rabbit in a toga, while a previously dosed rat retches in the background. Despite its grotesque images, it is perhaps the most elaborate book of its kind from the gift book era.

56. Henry D. Moore: *The Winter Bloom.* Philadelphia: Hogan & Thompson, 1850.

Color-printed wood engravings

This literary gift book is notable for its plates printed from multiple woodblocks, in what the publisher called "the highest style of art with recent and original improvements." It is one of the very few instances in American gift books of printing multiple woodcut blocks in colors, with as many as seven different color blocks used in one instance. While the printing work is carefully done, with good registration, its overall quality was not sufficient to rival the evolving chromolithographic mediums. The publisher added an extra touch to this volume by printing the introductory material in red.

57. Mrs. S. T. Martyn, ed.: *The Ladies Wreath or Illustrated Annual.* New York: Martyn & Miller, 1850.

Hand-colored lithograph

Many of the less well done gift and literary annuals included color plates with a melange of other illustrations, gathered almost randomly. Mrs. Martyn, who issued an annual in 1848, 1849, and 1850, included numerous plates which look as if they were bought as remainders. In this volume, crude hand-colored lithographs of flowers are juxtaposed with steel plate engravings from Bartlett's *American Scenery,* woodcuts, and mezzotints. Only a few bear any relationship to the equally grab-bag text.

58. Rev. Henry Harbaugh: *The Birds of the Bible.* Philadelphia: Lindsay & Blakiston, [1854].

Chromolithograph

Books with spiritual or biblical themes were ideal as gift books. The Philadelphia lithographer, Thomas Sinclair, executed the chromolithographic plates for this book, using nine different stones on the elaborately detailed title page.

59. Eliza Craufurd Ball: *The Christian Armour.* New York: Charles Scribners, 1866.

Chromolithograph

Devotional books were popular candidates for extra-illustration in color. Ball's collection of religious poems was illuminated with elaborate border and title decoration executed by the New York firm of Major and Knapp, a successor firm to the famous lithography establishment of Sarony and Major. The five different stones used on the title page are skillfully combined for rich effect, which stems from juxtaposition of strong colors rather than any mixture through overprinting. This is perhaps the most sumptuous American devotional book of the era, with a lavishly stamped binding to match.

60. Lida Clarkson: *Indian Summer. Autumn Poems and Sketches.* New York: E. P. Dutton & Company, 1883.

Chromolithograph

Although the great age of the gift books was before the Civil War, the genre lived on in the 1870s and 1880s, generally illustrated with chromolithographs

59. Ball, *The Christian Armour.* Chromolithograph.

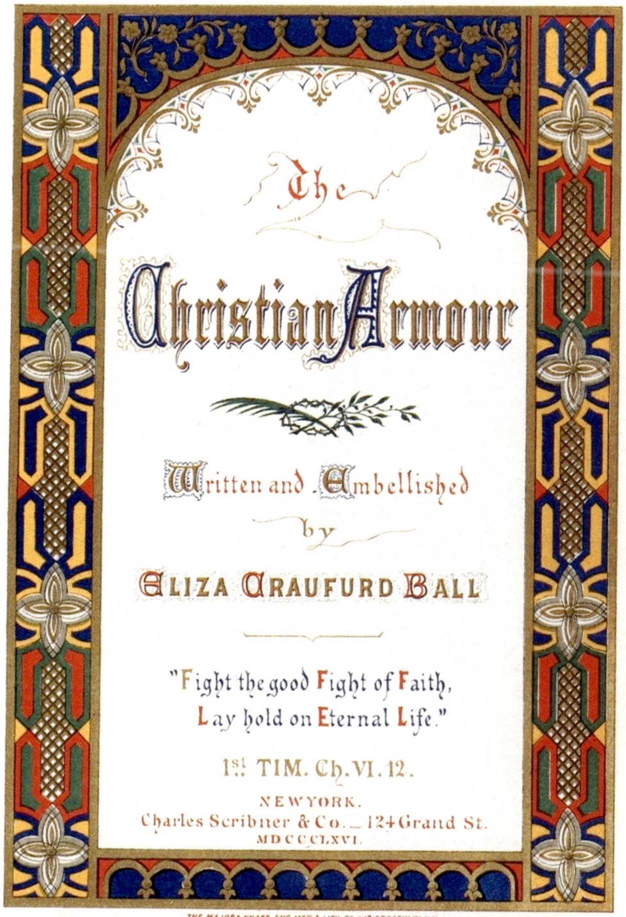

on botanical themes combined with poetry. The artist, Lida Clarkson, who also published works on home decoration and art instruction, produced a clutch of similar volumes. The heavy inking and rather oily colors were a deliberate effort to imitate the look of oil painting.

61. Eleanor W. Talbot: *My Lady's Casket of Jewels and Flowers for her Adorning.* Boston: Lee & Shepard, 1885.

Chromolithograph

The concept of a gift book which revealed real virtues evolved Imbert's *American Toilet* in the 1820s to this more elaborate chromolithographic version in the 1880s. "A Mixture Which Gives Sweetness to the Voice," when the folding flaps of the page are opened, is found to be "gentleness & sympathy." The Japanese look of the cabinet lends the air of prevailing fashion.

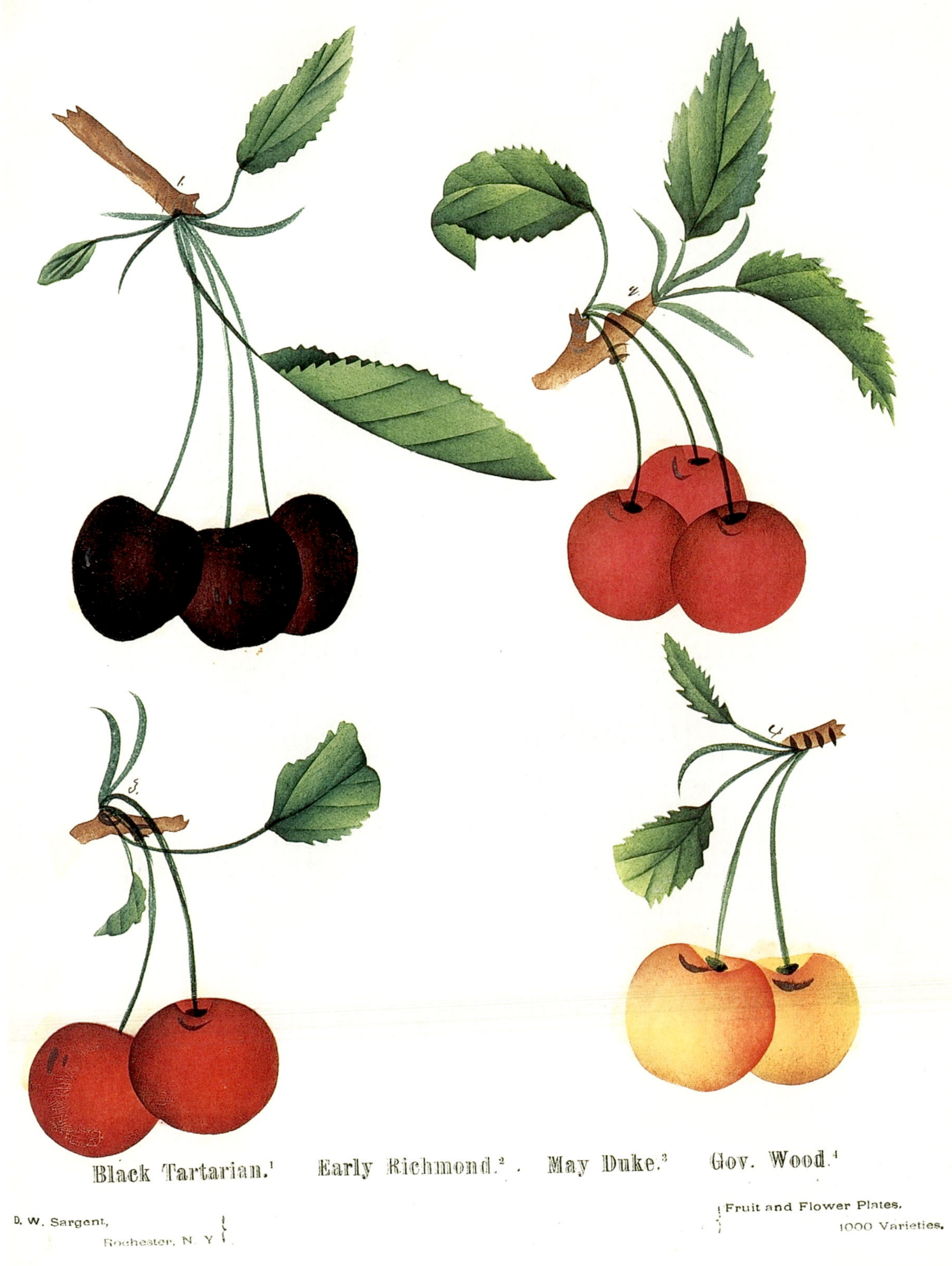

70. [Sargent], *The Specimen Book of Fruits....*
Stencil and hand coloring.

CASE 6: House and Home 1860–1890

An increasingly comfortable American middle and upper-middle class were eager to be instructed in how to house themselves, decorate their homes, and improve their grounds. Color plates became an important part of architecture books in the 1850s, illustrating styles of houses and how to paint them. Interior decoration, as heavily dependent on European models as fashion in clothing, was not taken up by American publishers until after the Civil War. Landscape design, on the other hand, followed very American models.

In Rochester, New York, a remarkable local industry sprang up around the need to illustrate sales catalogues for the fruits and flowers grown in the region's burgeoning nursery businesses. The color plates produced in Rochester up to the 1870s were largely produced by stencil and hand coloring, and are particularly appealing as a form of folk art. Later in the century, chromolithography replaced these earlier forms, as it displaced most hand coloring from book illustration.

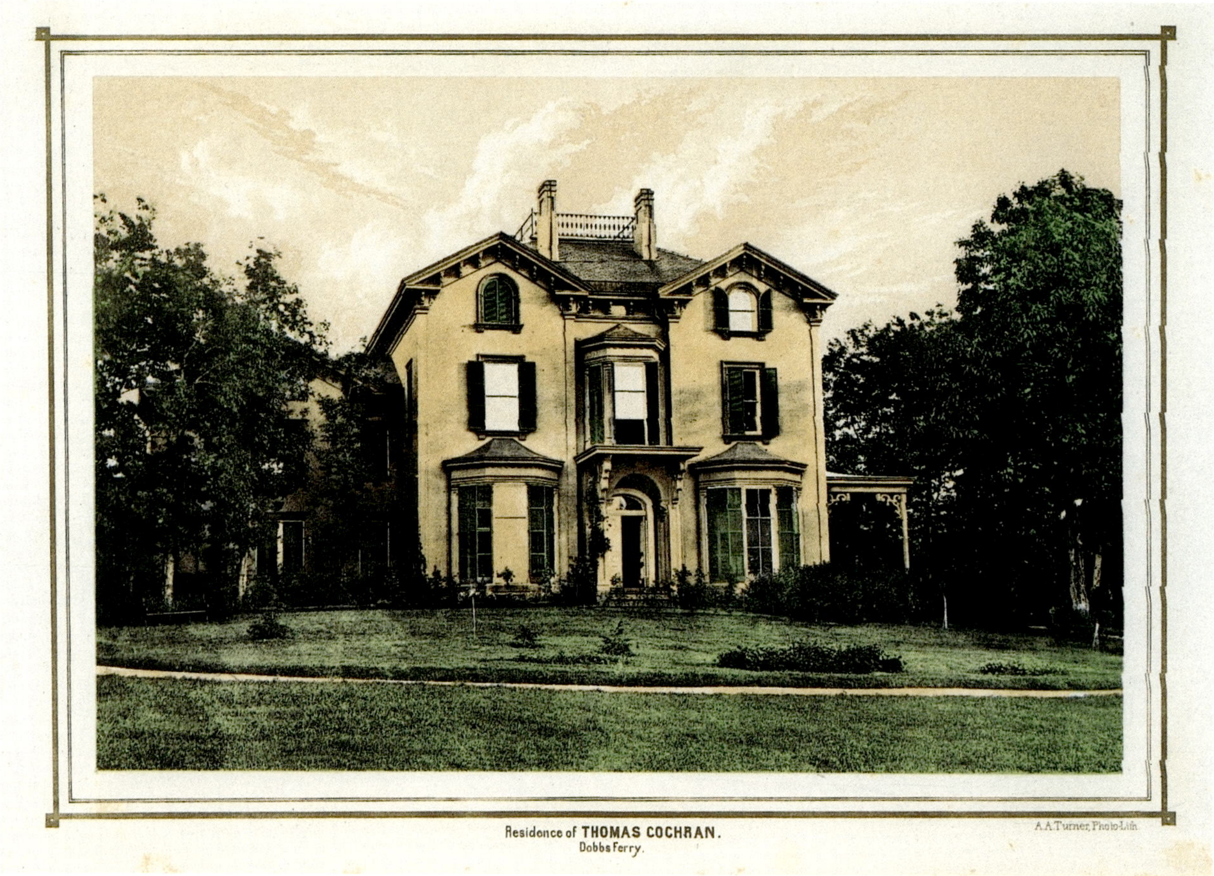

62. Turner,
Villas on the Hudson.
Tinted photolithograph
colored with stencil blocks.

62. A. A. Turner: *Villas on the Hudson. A Collection of Photo-Lithographs of Thirty-one Country Residences.* New York: D. Appleton, 1860.

Tinted photolithograph colored with stencil blocks

This book is generally considered to be the first large-scale use of photolithography in America. The plates are based on photographs by Turner taken in 1858 and 1859, illustrating the vacation homes of wealthy New Yorkers who had built themselves pleasure palaces from Fordham north to Tarrytown. These lavish villas, often with whimsical architectural features, remind us that the excesses of the Hamptons in modern times had their 19th-century rivals. The plates were colored with brown and green stencil on top of the tinted photolithograph, creating a remarkable visual effect.

63. Samuel Sloan: *The Model Architect. A Series of Original Designs for Cottages, Villas, Suburban Residences, etc.*

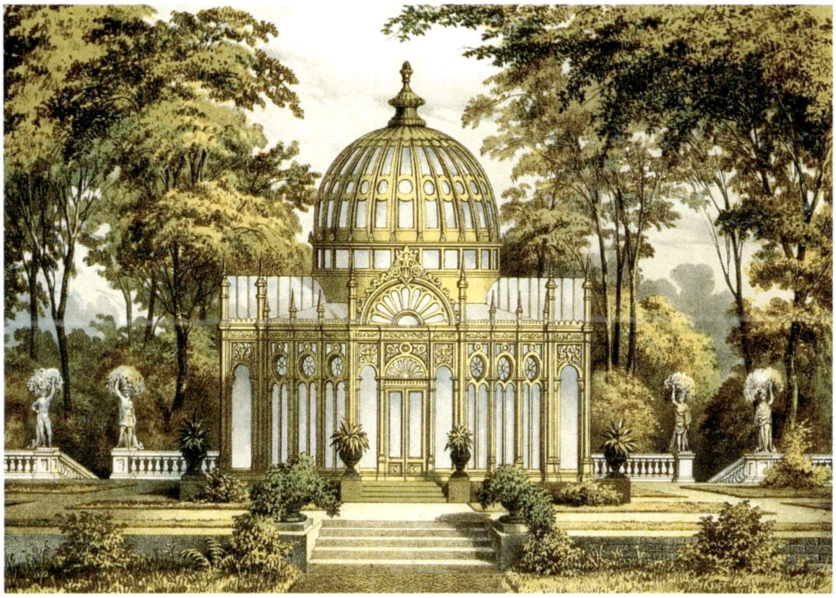

63. Sloan,
The Model Architect. . . .
Chromolithograph.

Accompanied by Explanations, Specifications, Estimates, and Elaborate Details. Philadelphia: J. B. Lippincott & Co., 1868.

Chromolithograph

Architectural pattern books published in the United States, which inevitably had a large number of plates, were almost entirely devoid of color before 1850. The prolific architect, Samuel Sloan, changed this with a number of influential works on architectural design in the 1850s and 1860s. Sloan's books were filled with tinted and colored lithographs showing exterior and interior designs for houses in an eclectic range of styles from Gothic to Oriental via Italianate. He offered not only design patterns and floor plans, but estimated costs and provided interior decoration ideas as well. Colored illustrations played an important part in Sloan's campaign to improve the architectural tastes of the expanding middle class.

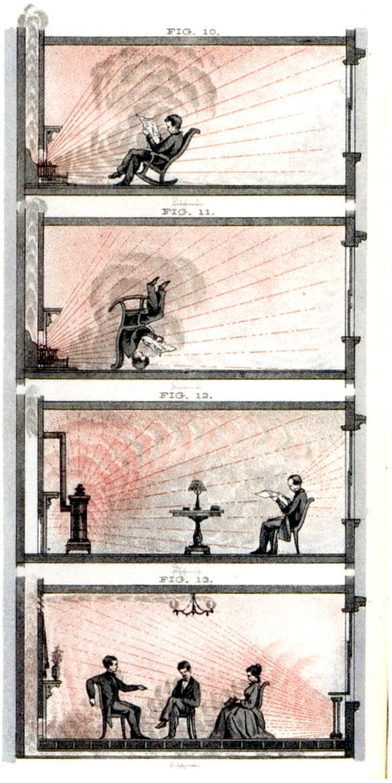

64. Leeds,
Lectures on Ventilation.
Chromolithograph.

64. Lewis W. Leeds: *Lectures on Ventilation.* New York: John Wiley & Sons, 1876.

Tinted lithograph

Leeds was an early crusader for the scientific ventilation of buildings, believing that most people were being poisoned by the heating and lighting systems in their homes and work places. He illustrated his pioneering notions on how to avoid such problems with a series of original and amusing plates showing the flow of heat and smoke.

65. Charles L. Eastlake: *Hints on Household Taste in Furniture, Upholstery, and other Details.* Boston: James R. Osgood and Company, 1877.

Chromolithograph

American publishers continually drew on European design sources, especially in interior decoration. Eastlake's highly influential work was first published in London in 1868, and went through many English and American editions. He was an advocate of the Aesthetic Movement, proposing more practical and less cluttered designs than the high Victorian taste then in fashion. Besides chromolithographs of floor design patterns, the illustrations include color-printed textured wallpaper samples.

66. Dr. J. Von Falke: Charles C. Perkins, trans.: *Art in the House. Historical, Critical, and Aesthetical Studies on the Decoration and Furnishing of the Dwelling.* Boston: Louis Prang, 1879.

Chromolithograph

By the time Louis Prang issued this American edition of Van Falke's study of grand homes through the ages, an increasingly comfortable American audience could take an interest in the history of luxury housing. Chromolithographs were juxtaposed as highlights of color in a text which also employed albertypes, steel cuts, and woodcuts. Prang was already capable of the remarkable control of color which made him the greatest printer of chromolithography in the United States during its golden era, the last quarter of the 19th century.

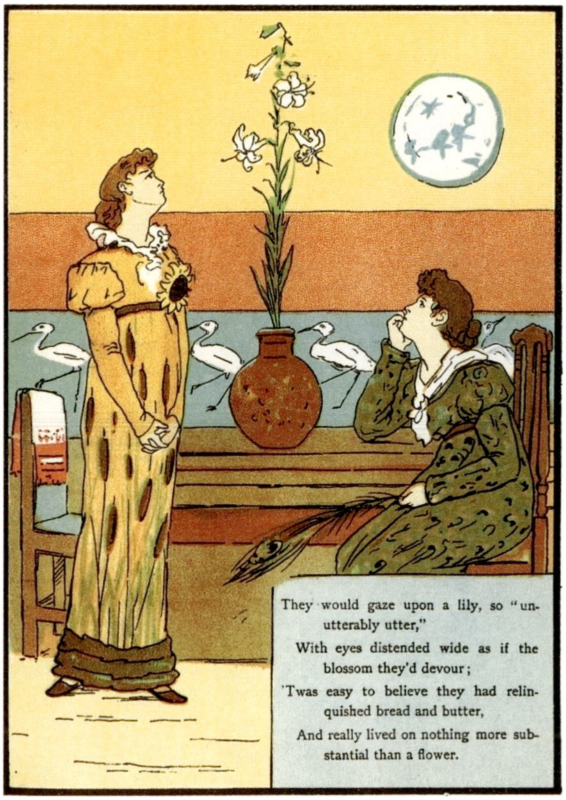

67. Josephine Pollard: *The Decorative Sisters. A Modern Ballad... with Illustrations by Walter Satterlee.* New York: A. D. F. Randolph and Co., 1881.

Chromolithograph

By 1881, some Americans had heard enough instruction from the Aesthetic Movement. This amusing work, executed entirely in chromolithography after the artist, Walter Satterlee, is a gentle spoof on the earnest home decoration ideas expounded by its devotees. The "decorative sisters," Dorothea and Dorinda, are lured from rural simplicity by a visiting landscape painter, and soon fill their house with painted vases, peacock feathers, lilies, and stenciled wallpaper. The accompanying poem describes them: "The Decorative Sisters were so mystically mystic, – / So whimiscally whimsey – so intensively intense – / That those who did not know 'twas Aesthetic and Artistic, / Would surely think that neither had a grain of common sense."

68. [Lucas and Co.], *Modern House Painting Designs.* Chromolithograph.

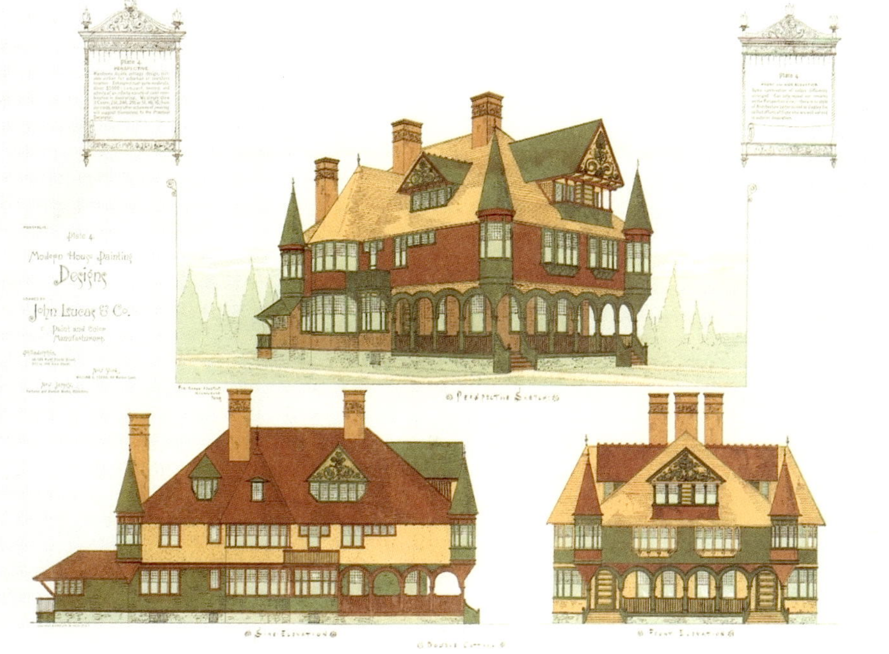

67. Pollard, *The Decorative Sisters.* Chromolithograph.

68. [John Lucas and Co.]: *Modern House Painting Designs.* New York: John Lucas and Co., 1887.

Chromolithograph

In the 1880s paint companies such as Lucas, Devoe, Seeley Brothers, and Sherwin-Williams produced a number of lavish portfolios of painting designs for buildings. These fall somewhere between books and trade catalogues, intended to promote products and provide design ideas. Lucas' catalogue is the most elaborate of such publications, illustrated with thirty plates of potential color choices and architectural designs for houses, barns, churches, cottages, and town halls.

69. J. Weidenmann: *Beautifying Country Homes. A Handbook of Landscape Gardening. Illustrated by Plans of Places Already Improved.* New York: Orange Judd, 1870.

Chromolithograph

Color plates could reinforce design ideas far more effectively than other forms of illustration. Weidenmann began his career as the superintendent of Cedar Hill Cemetery in Hartford, a suburban burial ground with limited monuments and extensive landscaping. From there he migrated to landscape design for homes, showing himself to be a disciple of A. J. Downing and Frederic Law Olmsted. This book illustrates the ground plans for a series of real and theoretical estates, showing buildings, grounds, plantings, and outbuildings in bold chromolithographs by H. Bencke, a New York lithographer.

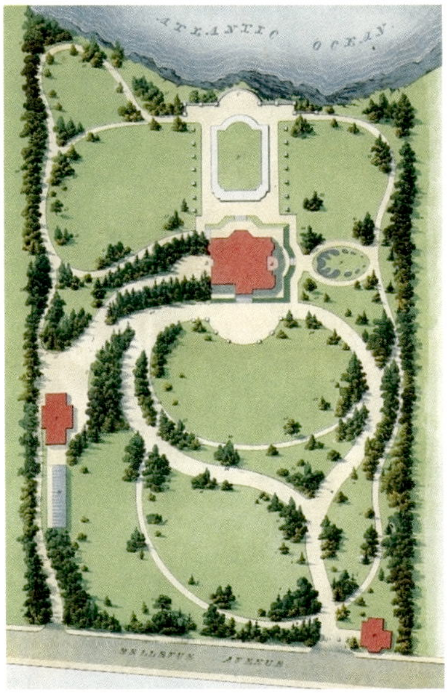

69. Weidenmann, *Beautifying Country Homes....* Chromolithograph.

70. [D. W. Sargent]: *The Specimen Book of Fruits, Flowers and Ornamental Trees, Carefully Drawn & Colored from Nature for the Use of Nurserymen.* Rochester, N. Y.: D. W. Sargent, [ca. 1865].

Stencil and hand coloring

The color plate industry in Rochester, New York, has a unique history. In the 1840s the city became a leading center of the nursery business, especially fruit trees. To advertise their products to customers around the country, the growers turned to a local bookseller, D. M. Dewey, who began to produce plates illustrating various species for sale. Dewey's first plates were issued in the 1850s, and he was soon joined by D. W. Sargent and others. In the early period the plates were usually produced by stencil and hand coloring, as in this Sargent album. Chromolithography gradually replaced the hand-finished plates and became the primary medium by the mid-1880s.

71. Franklin Reuben Elliott: *Hand Book of Practical Landscape Gardening Designed for City and Suburban Residences, and Country School-Houses, Containing Designs for Lots and Grounds.* Rochester: D. M. Dewey, Horticultural Books, 1877.

Chromolithograph

This thoroughly practical work, aimed at "the plain, common-sense man," was far more modest in its plans than Weidenmann's estates. Elliott argued that there was pleasure to be gained by planned planting, as well as increasing the value of the home in the real estate market. The book is thrifty in its makeup, since the publisher, Dewey, used leftover plates manufactured for nursery catalogues in 1872 as illustrations in this 1877 imprint. Keyed maps in the books showed the user exactly where to plant which trees. Such instruction was undoubtedly helpful to Dewey's main customers, the nursery owners.

72. [Stecher Lithographic Company]: [*Album of Fruit and Flower Plates*]. Rochester: Stecher Lithographic Company, [ca. 1890].

Chromolithograph

As the Rochester printing industry blossomed, collections of plates illustrating fruits and plants for sale became an indispensable reference for nurseries around the country. Such books were generally made up of loose plates to suit the individual firm, often mixing work from different printers such as Dewey, Sargent, and Stecher, or ones executed in different mediums. As a result, virtually every album is unique in its makeup. Elaborate sales books were produced which could be opened to show a number of different varieties at once, as in this example. The most elaborate foldouts could show up to fifty plates at once.

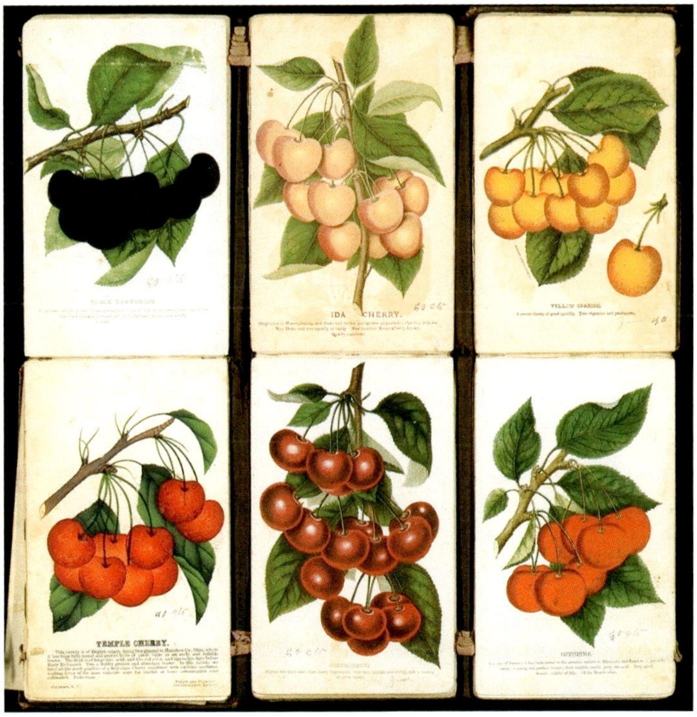

72. [Stecher Lithographic Company], [*Album of Fruit and Flower Plates*]. Chromolithograph.

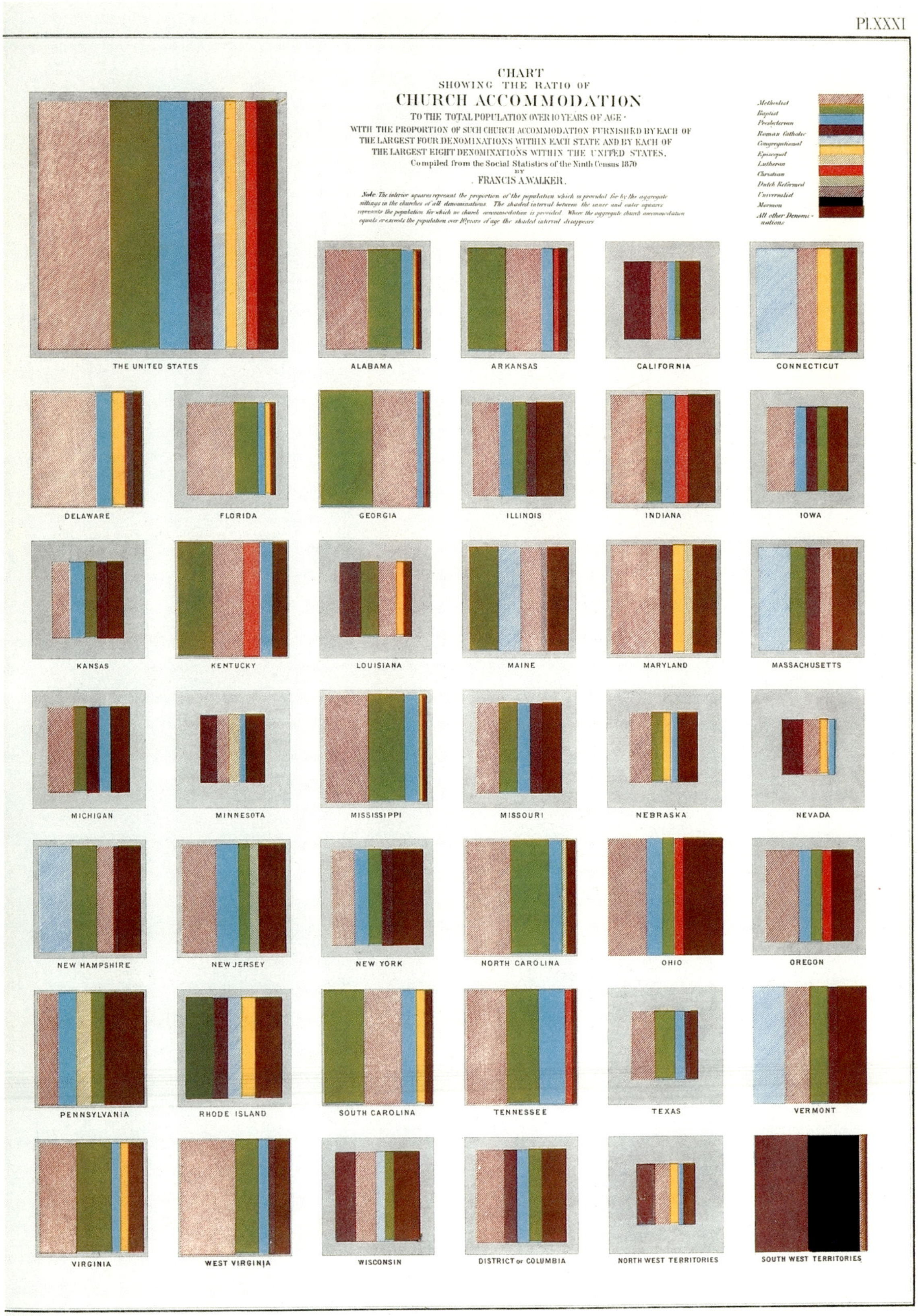

84. [Walker], *Statistical Atlas of the United States....*
Chromolithograph.

CASE 7: Color in the Aid of Science 1825–1880

Evolving fields of science and medicine found color plates an important means of conveying exact information. The detection of diseases and surgical education, for example, were greatly aided by illustration in medical works. From the 1840s, government support for scientific investigation became a major factor in the funding of color illustration in books. The publication of national scientific surveys, beginning with the findings of the Wilkes Expedition in the late 1840s, became an entire industry by the time the results of the Pacific Railroad Surveys were being published a decade later. These were hugely expensive (and hotly debated) government expenditures at the time, producing literally millions of plates. Although such government funding was more modest after the Civil War, the role of official projects in supporting color printing remained significant.

Color also began to be used as a way of conveying quantitative information. These innovative plates prefigure methods of displaying data which have become commonplace, but were revolutionary at the time.

73. James Ellsworth DeKay [et al]: *Natural History of New York.* Albany: Carroll & Cook, Printers to the Assembly [and others], 1842–1895.

Hand-colored lithograph

The *Natural History of New York* was the first major scientific survey in the United States to be underwritten by government funding. Begun in 1836 under the direction of James DeKay, the project was published in six series covering Zoology, Botany, Mineralogy, Geology, Agriculture, and Paleontology. Most of the thirty volumes in the series were published in 1842–1844, although the last two sections were not completed until 1894. Hand-colored lithographs lavishly illustrate the first four sections, with almost five hundred plates ranging from depictions of individual species to large folding panoramas in the Geology segment.

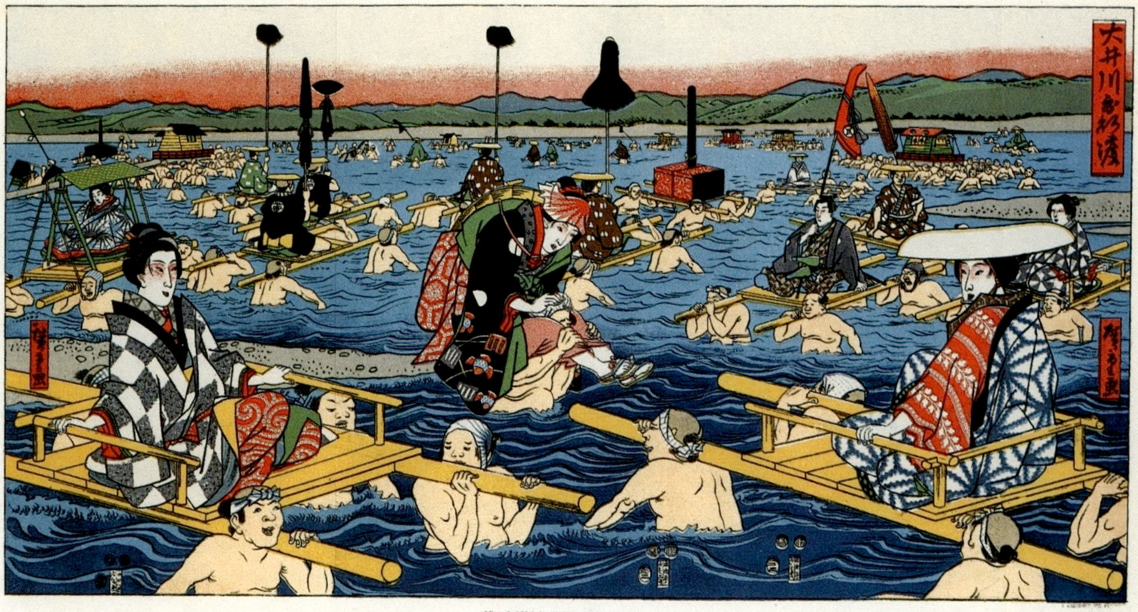

CROSSING THE OHO-E-GA-WA.
[Province Suruga]

74. [Matthew C. Perry]: Francis L. Hawks, comp.: *Narrative of the Expedition of an American Squadron to the China Seas and Japan, Performed in the Years 1852, 1853, and 1854, Under the Command of Commodore*

M. C. Perry, United States Navy, by Order of the Government of the United States.... Washington: A. O. P. Nicholson, Printer, 1856.

Tinted lithograph

Commodore Perry's famous expedition to open Japan to the West formed the basis for a lavish government publication combining a narrative of the events in Japan with scientific data gathered en route. The chromolithographs illustrating the narrative were based partially on the drawings of William Heine (who independently published a lavish folio, *Graphic Scenes of the Japan Expedition*, New York, 1856) and partially on daguerreotypes by Eliphalet Brown, Jr. These plates are an early instance of a daguerreotype being used as the basis for a lithograph, and the final results have a strikingly "photographic" quality to them. Shown in the exhibition are plates executed by two different lithographers: Peter S. Duval (on the left) chose to use shades of brown as a tint, while Thomas Sinclair (on the right) used green and brown tints.

74. [Perry], *Narrative of the Expedition... to the China Seas...*
Chromolithograph.

75. [Pacific Railroad Surveys]: *Reports of Explorations and Surveys, to Ascertain the Most Practicable and Economical Route for a Railroad from the Mississippi River to the Pacific Ocean. Made Under the Direction of the Secretary of War, in 1853–4....* Washington: Beverley Tucker, Printer, 1855–1860.

Tinted lithograph with hand coloring

The Pacific Railroad Surveys of the 1850s, undertaken to determine possible routes for a transcontinental railroad, were the vehicles for the most extensive scientific studies of the 19th century funded by the U.S. government. The geography, geology, and natural history of the American West was exhaustively investigated in a series of expeditions, and the results were published in a thirteen-volume set containing hundreds of hand-colored lithographs and chromolithographs, as well as steel cuts and woodcuts. It is estimated that a total of twenty-one million plates (both colored and uncolored) by different New York and Philadelphia firms were produced for the series between 1855 and 1860. In sheer numbers, it was the greatest printing project of the century.

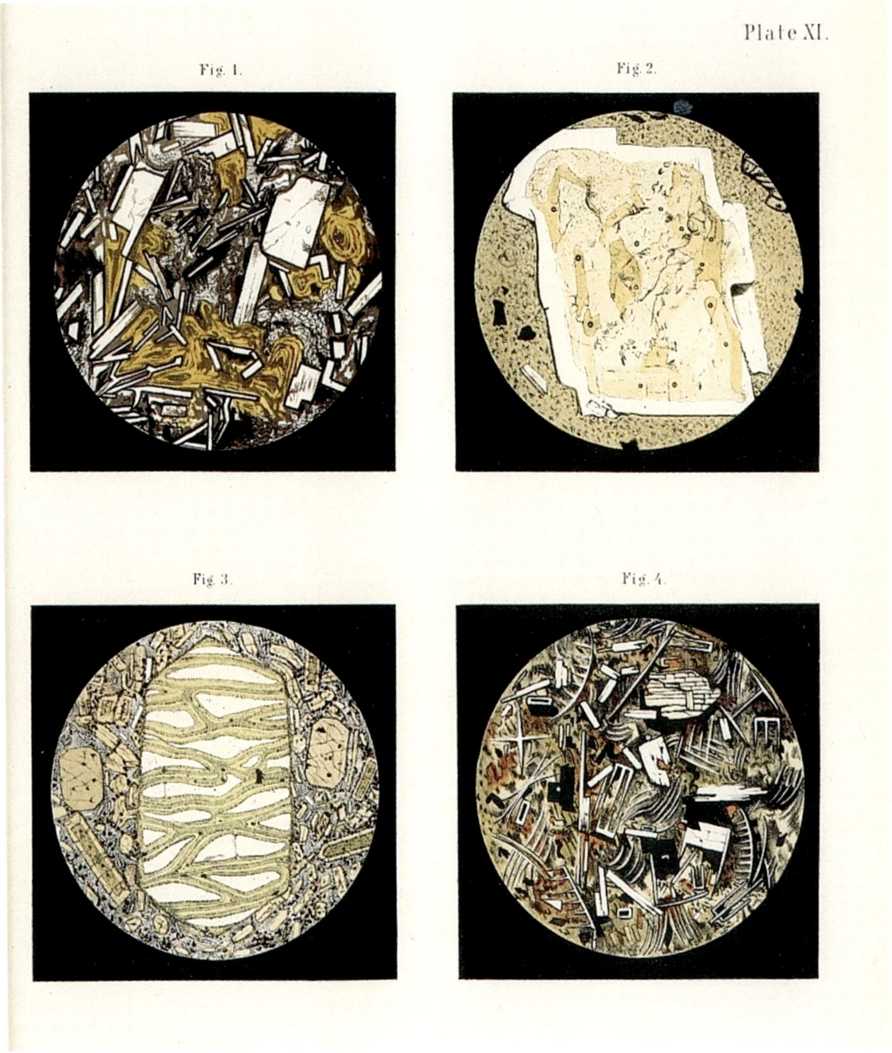

76. King, *Report of the Geological Exploration....* Chromolithograph.

76. [Clarence King, et al]: *Report of the Geological Exploration of the Fortieth Parallel Made by Order of the Secretary of War....* Washington: Government Printing Office, 1870–1880.

Chromolithograph

After the Civil War the U. S. Government continued its patronage of science and surveying in the American West with the King, Hayden, Powell, and Wheeler surveys. Clarence King, dubbed "the best and the brightest of his generation" by his friend, Henry Adams, conducted the survey across the 40th Parallel. The publication of the results includes the usual maps and views, but also features chromolithographic representations of microscopic cross-sections, using the medium to focus on a purely scientific illustration divorced from the narrative or topographical studies.

77. Benjamin Travers: *A Synopsis of the Diseases of the Eye, and Their Treatment; to Which Are Prefixed a Short Anatomical Description and a Sketch of the Physiology of That Organ.* New York: E. Bliss, E. White, 1825.

Hand-colored engraving

Color was often a vital component of medical illustration, and some of the most lavish use of color in scientific publications of the 19th century appears in medical books. Because of their often unappealing subject matter, they have been largely ignored by bibliographers of American illustrated works. Whitman Bennett called them "essentially repulsive." Careful and accurate color illustrations were important to medical education, however, and the engraver, Peter Maverick, took the greatest care with these plates.

78. George Spratt: *Obstetric Tables; Comprising Graphic Illustrations, with Descriptions and Practical Remarks; Exhibiting on Dissected Plates Many Important Aspects of Midwifery. First American Edition, from the Fourth and Greatly Improved London Edition.* Philadelphia: James A. Bill, 1850.

Hand-colored lithograph

Copied from the London original, this book contains many plates with complex overlays of movable flaps to illustrate anatomy. The American editor states in the preface: "It was so novel and so difficult a piece of work, that no lithographers liked to undertake it…the Editor, however, having some similar work done by Messrs. Wagner & McGuigan, was convinced from what he saw of their skill, that it could be done by them fully equal to the original, and much cheaper." The plates have up to five levels of hinged flaps, showing details of progressive stages of gestation or medical procedures during birth. Wagner & McGuigan was one of the leading Philadelphia lithographic firms at the time.

79. Joseph Pancoast: *A Treatise on Operative Surgery; Comprising a Description of the Various Processes of the Art, Including All the Operations….* Philadelphia: Published by A. Hart, 1852.

Hand-colored lithograph

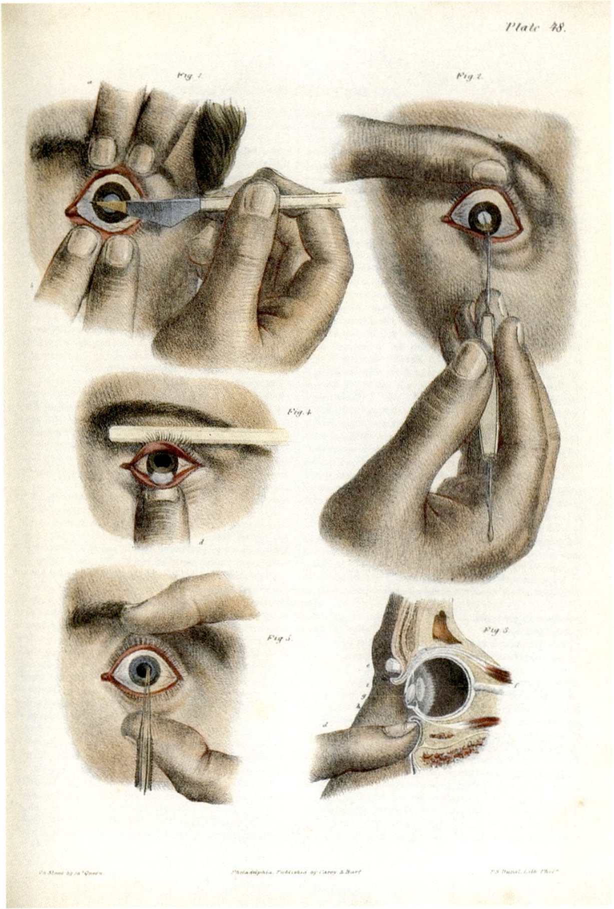

79. Pancoast, *A Treatise on Operative Surgery....* Hand-colored lithograph.

Pancoast's work was one of the most extensively illustrated medical works published in America before the Civil War. It was available with either uncolored or colored plates, and in the latter format it is one of the most impressive color plate books of its era. The plates illustrate a broad variety of surgical techniques, usually with multiple figures per sheet. Peter S. Duval was the lithographer.

80. [Joseph K. Barnes, ed.]: *The Medical and Surgical History of the War of the Rebellion....* Washington: Government Printing Office, 1875–1883.

Chromolithograph

The horrors of the Civil War provided surgeons with a multitude of complicated cases. This vast work, in six bulky volumes, attempted to quantify the medical knowledge so painfully gained, extensively illustrating case histories with chromolithographic plates. The set marked the first major government subsidy in publishing medical research, the only such official study to rival the expenditure made for exploration surveys of the era.

81. Eckardt, *An Atlas of Anatomy....* Chromolithograph.

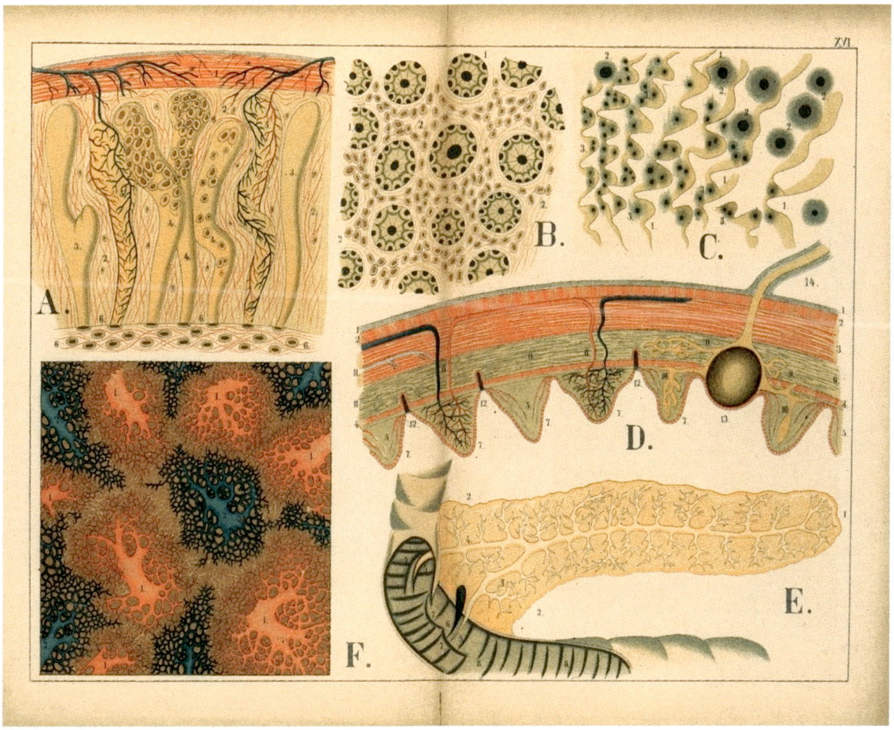

81. Theodore Eckardt: *An Atlas of Anatomy or the Human Body, in Twenty-four Color Plates.* Indianapolis: G. H. Keyler & Co., 1881.

Chromolithograph

After the Civil War the lower cost and widespread availability of chromolithography encouraged the manufacture of less expensive medical and scientific textbooks. This collection of plates advertised not only its low price, but its wide appeal, claiming itself to be useful not only to medical students and science teachers, but children as well. Its editor suggested it as "an acceptable gift to an intelligent youth of twelve or fourteen." Color illustration in science began to enter the realm of the popular with the advent of cheaper printing techniques.

82. Edward L. Youmans: *Chemical Atlas; or, the Chemistry of Familiar Objects: Exhibiting the General Principles of the Science in a Series of Beautifully Colored Diagrams, and Accompanied by Explanatory Essays....* New York: D. Appleton & Company, 1855.

Color-printed woodblock and hand coloring

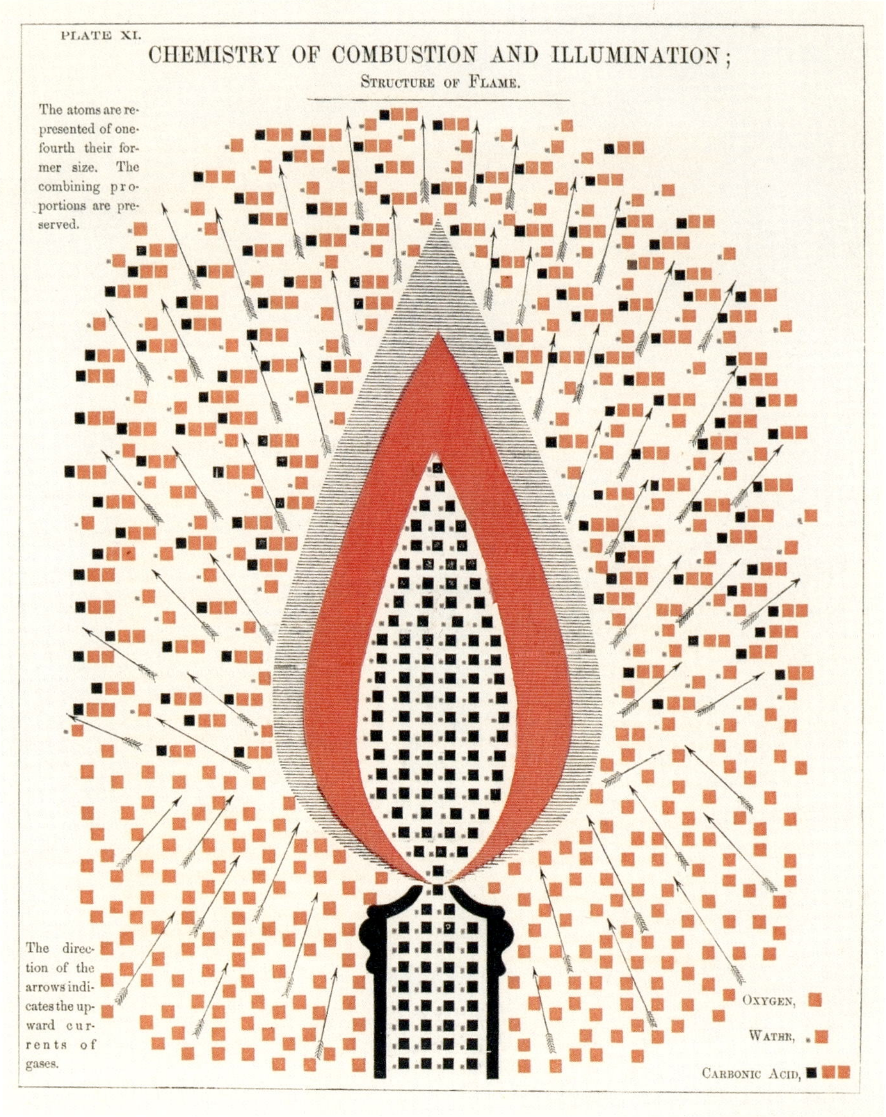

82. Youmans, *Chemical Atlas . . .* Color-printed woodblock and hand coloring.

This chemistry textbook was a pioneering publication in the use of color to convey quantitative information. Some plates display differing chemical elements with various colors, but the most striking illustration is that showing the chemical structure of a flame. Differing compounds are depicted with red, brown, and black printed blocks, finished by hand. The result is a striking and effective display of information.

83. E. W. Dimond: *The Chemistry of Combustion, Applied to the Economy of Fuel with Special Reference to the Construction of Fire Chambers, for Steam Boilers.* Worcester: Edward R. Fiske, 1867.

Chromotypograph

83. Dimond, *The Chemistry of Combustion…* Chromotypograph.

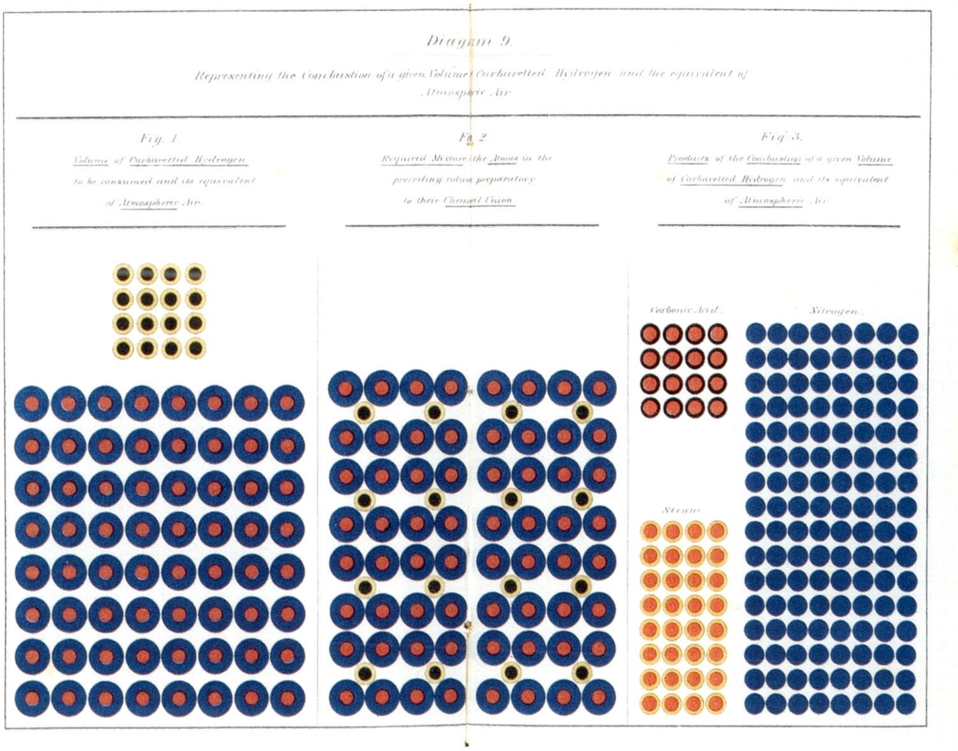

The author, an engineer, was concerned with discovering the most efficient methods of turning fuel into heat. He illustrates the mechanics of combustion with plates representing the chemical reactions involved using red, blue, black, and yellow in different combinations. The resulting plates, printed from metal relief blocks, effectively convey information, but also have an appealing abstract beauty.

84. [Francis A. Walker]: *Statistical Atlas of the United States Based on the Results of the Ninth Census 1870….* New York: Julius Bien, Lith., 1874.

Chromolithograph

The atlas volume to the Ninth United States Census, largely designed by its Director, Francis A. Walker, was an extraordinary departure in the display of information. Walker pioneered the use of tones and intensity of color to show population statistics ranging from the prevalence of disease to the density of crops. Perhaps his most dramatic plate, however, displays the religious affiliations of the United States and territories. Forty-one separate boxes contain strips of up to twelve colors coded by denomination, showing the percentage of affiliation, sect by sect. A staggering quantity of data is conveyed in a single folio sheet.

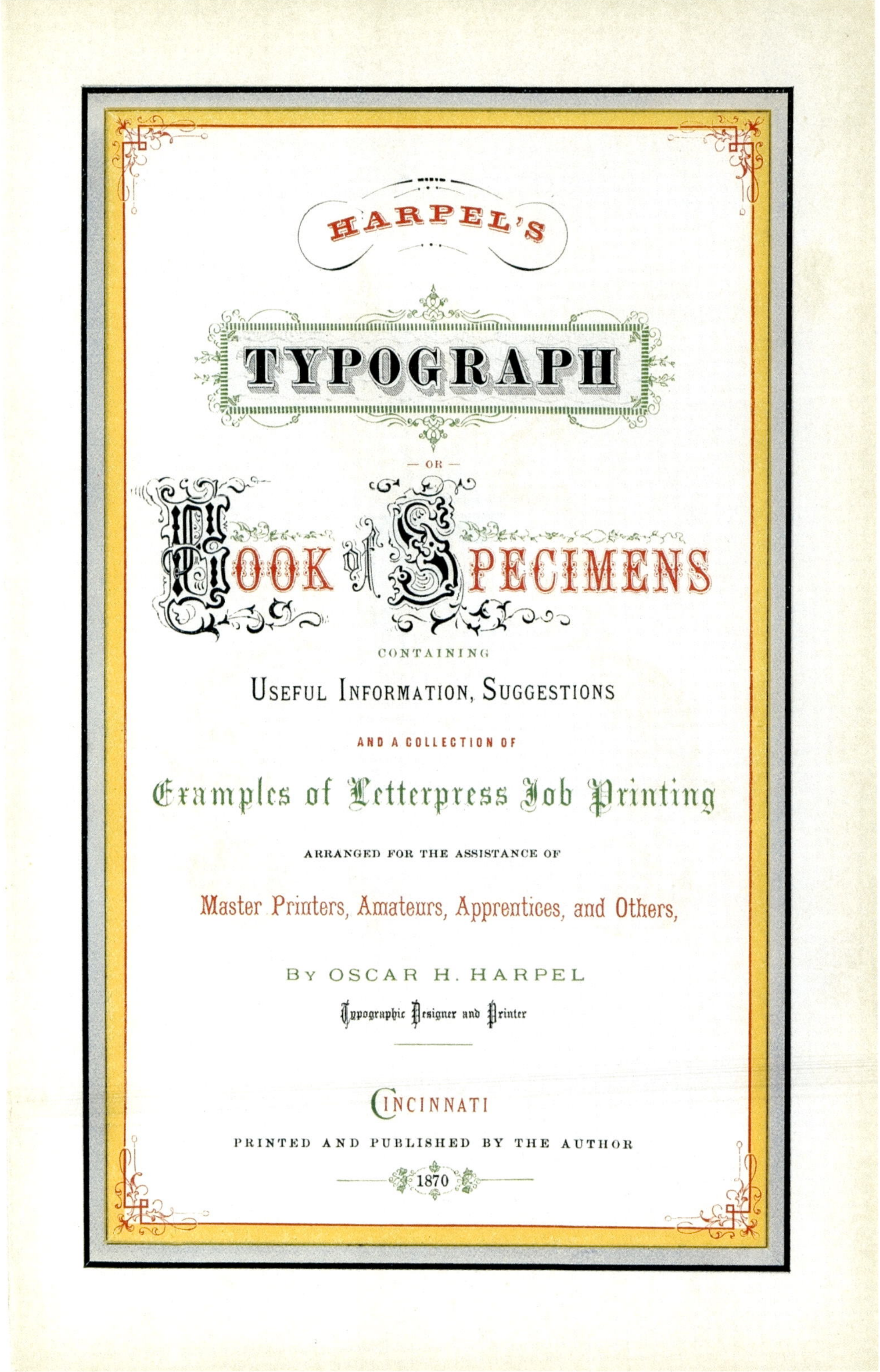
HARPEL'S

TYPOGRAPH

— OR —

BOOK of SPECIMENS

CONTAINING

USEFUL INFORMATION, SUGGESTIONS

AND A COLLECTION OF

Examples of Letterpress Job Printing

ARRANGED FOR THE ASSISTANCE OF

Master Printers, Amateurs, Apprentices, and Others,

BY OSCAR H. HARPEL

Typographic Designer and Printer

CINCINNATI

PRINTED AND PUBLISHED BY THE AUTHOR

1870

92. Harpel, *Harpel's Typograph....*
Electrotype and color printing from type and ornaments.

CASE 8: Exotica 1839–1886

Although the United States completely dominated the production of color plate books in the Western Hemisphere in the 19th century, interesting work was done in Canada, Mexico, the Caribbean, and South America. Examples are shown here, as well as a series of works from the United States unusual in their manner of execution. Also shown are several works of printing instruction intended to guide printers working in color.

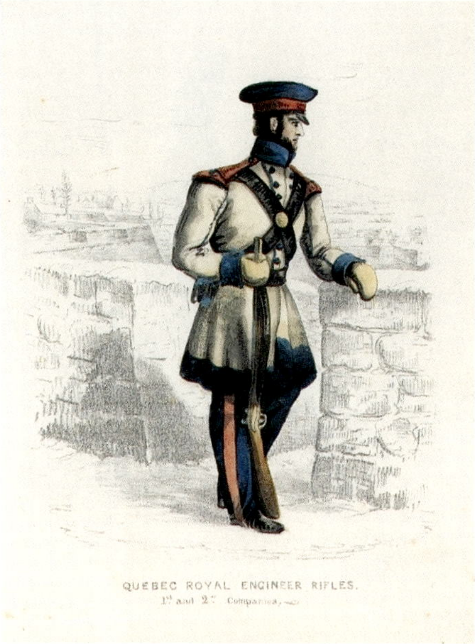

85. [Hope], *The Quebec Volunteers.*
Hand-colored lithograph.

85. [James Hope]: *The Quebec Volunteers.* Quebec: Printed and published by Peregrine Pouchbelt and Rodrick Ramrod, 1839.

Hand-colored lithograph

This anonymous production is the earliest Canadian color plate book. It illustrates the uniforms of different military units which served in Quebec during the abortive rebellion against British rule in 1837. The crudeness of the plates and partial nature of the coloring, as well as the jesting imprint, suggest this may have been an amateur project to while away a long winter, probably printed on the military press at Quebec. The artist is thought to have been Lieut.-Col. James Hope of the Coldstream Guards, although the lithographer is unidentified.

86. Ramon Torres Mendez: *Costumbres Neo-Granadinas.* Bogota: Martinez, 1851–1852.

Tinted lithograph with hand coloring

The history of lithography and color printing in South America has not been deeply investigated, but it is safe to say that it was limited to a few large cities, primarily the two with the closest maritime contact with Europe: Rio de Janeiro and Lima. However, this costume book from Colombia demonstrates that quite unexpected things can turn up. Standard bibliographies record the Paris edition of 1860, but fail to note the Bogota original of this costume book illustrating local types. Torres Mendez was trained as a printer by the very English sounding Bogota firm of Fox & Stokes, but was self-taught as an artist.

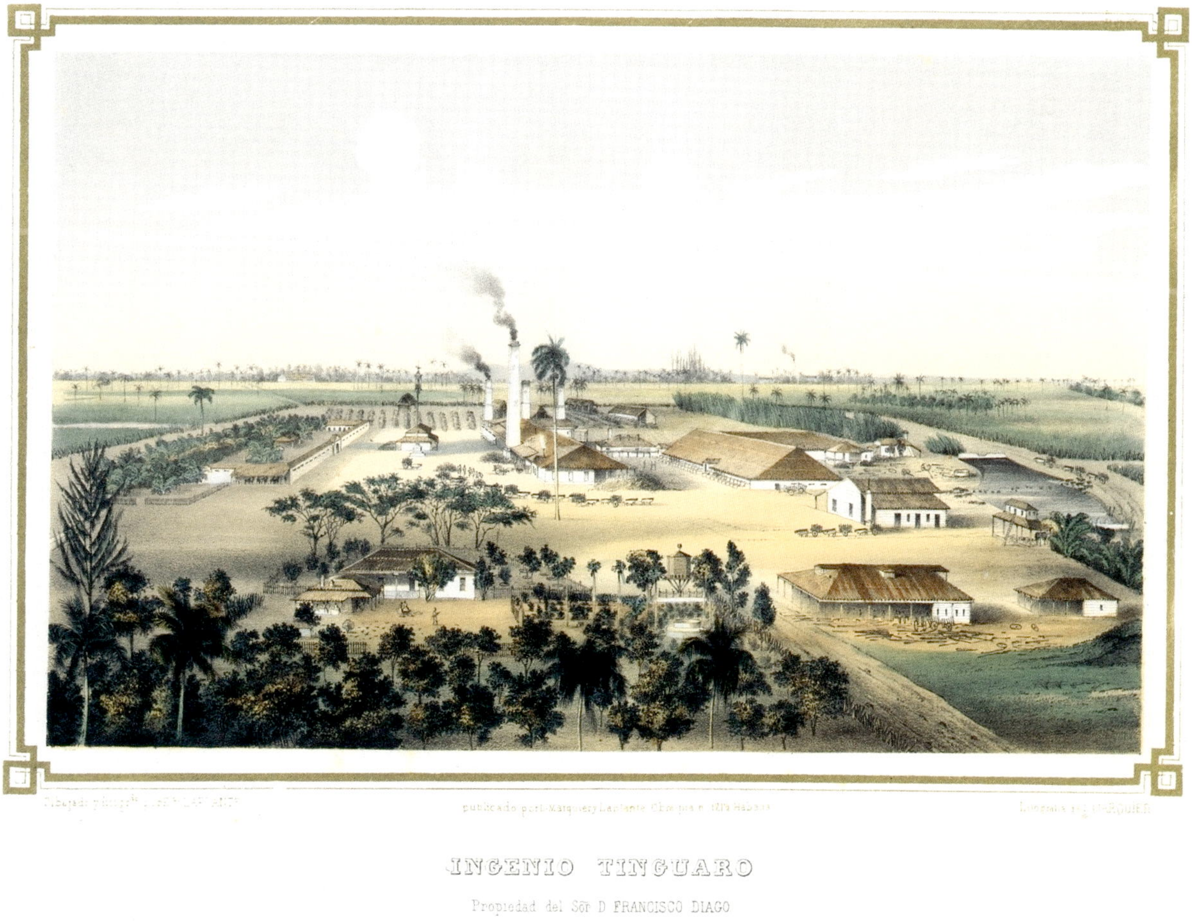

87. Cantero, *Los Ingenios....* Chromolithograph with hand coloring.

87. Justo German Cantero: *Los Ingenios: Coleccion de Vistas de la Principales Ingenios de Azucar de la Isla de Cuba....* Havana: Impreso en la lithografia de L. Marquier, 1857.

Chromolithograph with hand coloring

Outside of the United States, the best color printing work in the Americas in the 19th century was done in Havana. A work of natural history with engraved plates, sometimes found with contemporary color, had been produced there as early as 1787. The community of lithographers in the mid-19th century were primarily French immigrants, reflecting the Parisian tastes of the wealthy classes in Cuba. This book illustrates the major sugar estates of the island (the source of that wealth) in beautifully executed plates .

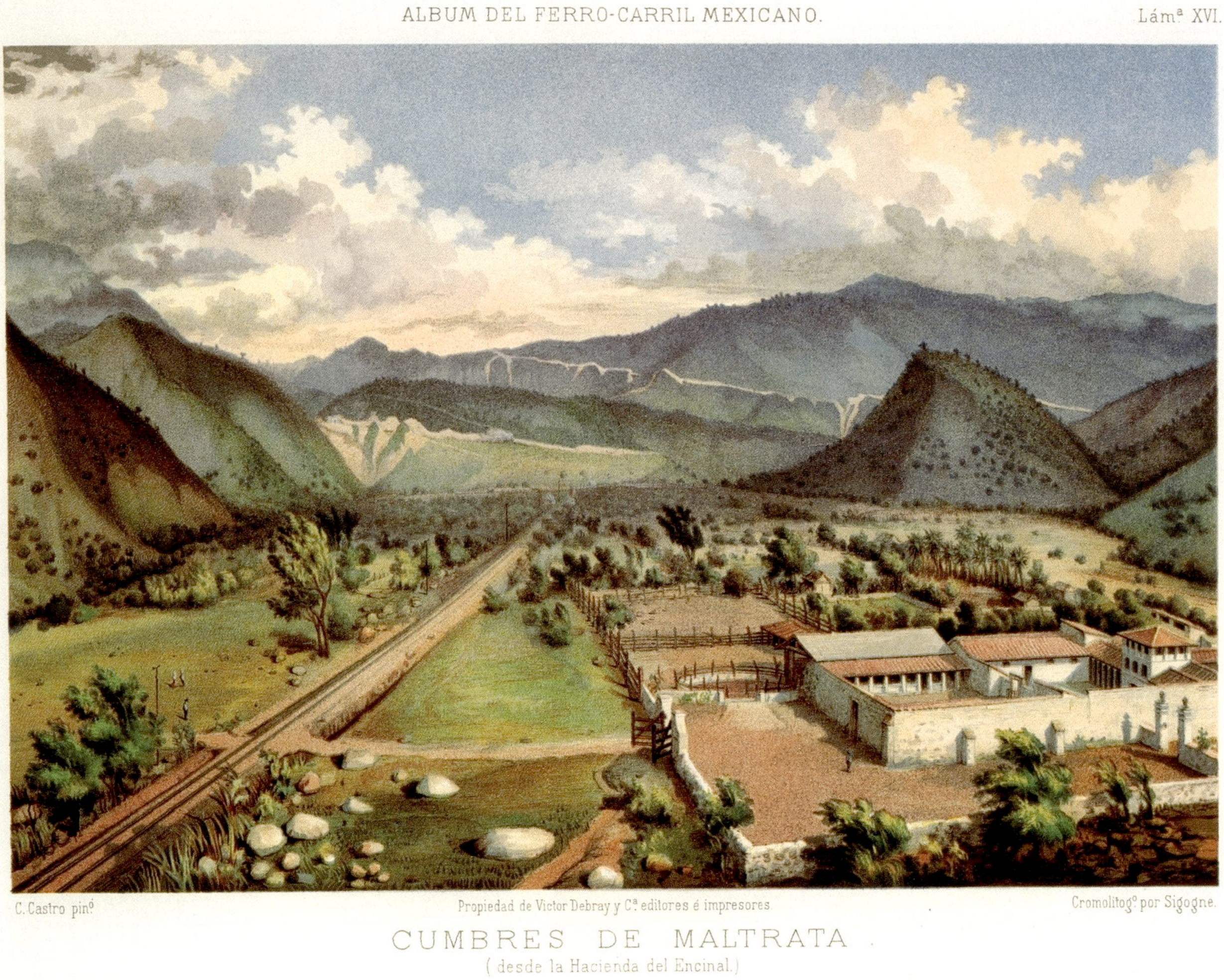

88. Castro and Cubas, *Album de Chemin de Fer Mexicano. . . .* Chromolithograph.

88. Casimio Castro and Antonio Garcia Cubas: *Album de Chemin de Fer Mexicano. . . .* Mexico: Victor Debray, 1877.

Chromolithograph

Mexico had a lively tradition of lithography from its beginnings there in 1826, most strikingly in monochrome political cartoon and caricature; however, relatively little color work was done there. The most notable and extravagant color plate book to appear was this history of the Veracruz-Mexico City railroad, illustrating scenes along its route. With text in Spanish, French, and English, and twenty-four plates in gaudy chromolithography, it was intended to encourage international investment.

89. T. W. Gwilt Mapleson: *Pearls of American Poetry Illuminated.* New York: Wiley and Putnam, [1853].

Chromolithograph

This collection of poems is one of the most elaborate examples of mimicking illuminated manuscripts by way of chromolithography. Printed on heavy card stock hinged into a binding, the volume combines the work of two different Philadelphia lithographers, Brett and Sinclair. Mapleson produced a string of similar books in the early 1850s, at the height of the gift book craze.

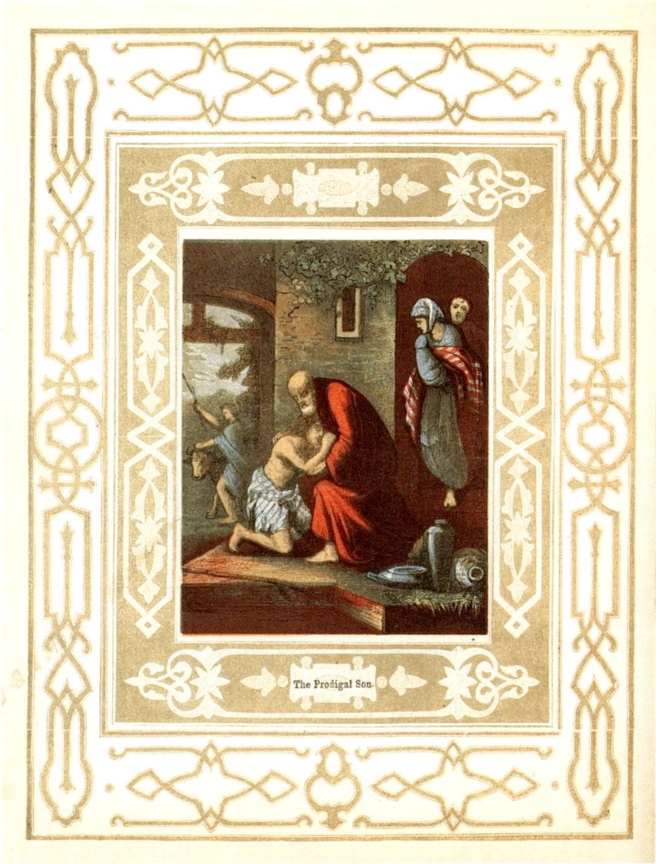

90. Kitto, *The Gallery of Scriptural Engravings. . . .* Chromoxylograph.

90. John Kitto: *The Gallery of Scriptural Engravings, Historical and Landscape, Printed in Oil Colors, from the Best Paintings of Raffaelle, Poussin, Correggio. . . .* Chicago: H. C. Foster, 1856.

Chromoxylograph

This book is something of a mystery, evidently pirated from the works of the English biblical scholar, John Kitto, who published numerous books of Bible illustrations in the 1830s and 1840s. The publisher, Foster, operated a Chicago bookstore, but he was not a printer, and no other book of this sort was produced in Chicago at such an early date. The method of color printing used (multiple impressions from wood blocks) was not widely practiced in American books of this period. It may be that the letterpress part of the book was produced in Chicago and the plates were imported from the East or Europe. On the other hand, given the importance of immigrants in every stage of 19th-century American color printing, a craftsman newly arrived in Chicago may have executed them there.

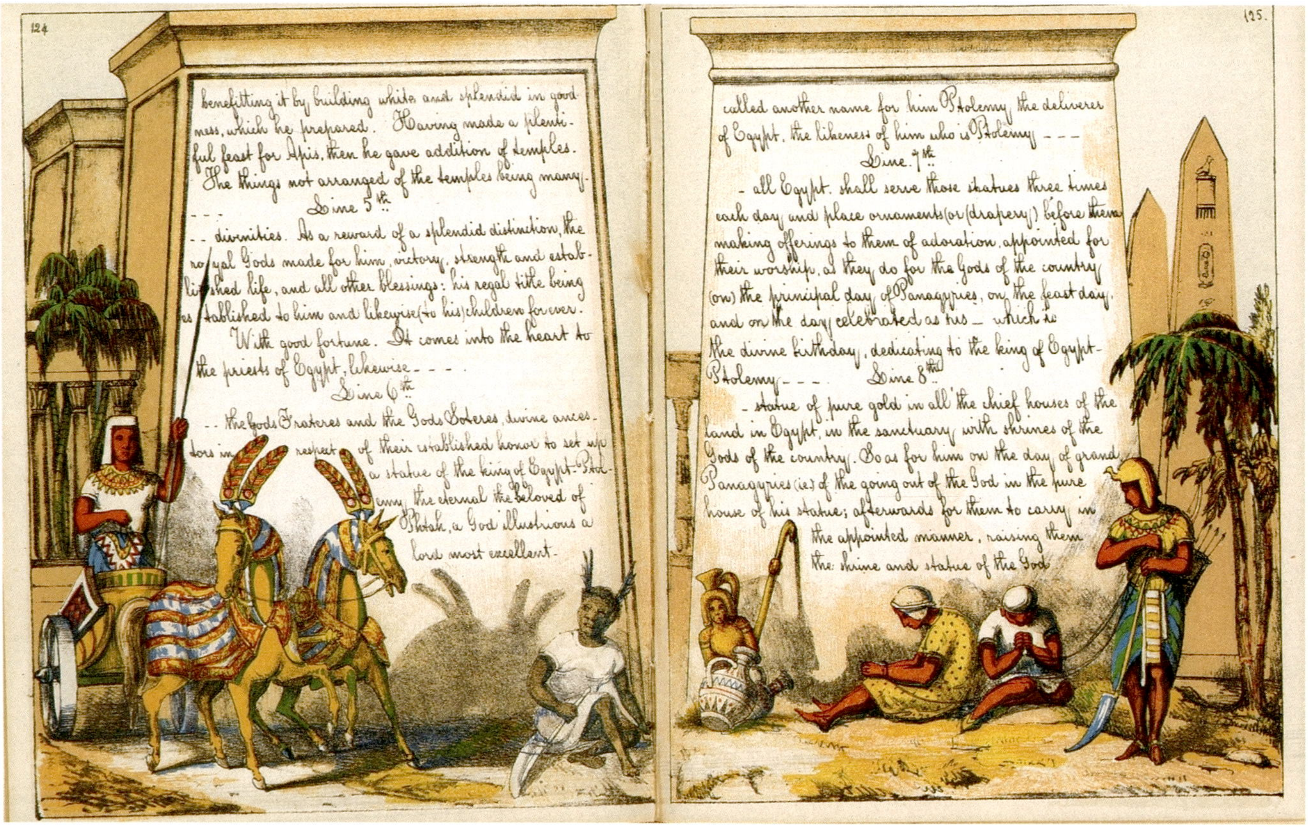
124

benefitting it by building white and splendid in goodness, which he prepared. Having made a plentiful feast for Apis, then he gave addition of temples. The things not arranged of the temples being many.

Line 5th.

- - - divinities. As a reward of a splendid distinction, the royal Gods made for him, victory, strength and established life, and all other blessings: his regal title being established to him and likewise (to his) children forever. With good fortune. It comes into the heart to the priests of Egypt, likewise - - -

Line 6th.

- - the Gods Fraters and the Gods Soteres, divine ancestors in respect of their established honor to set up a statue of the king of Egypt - Ptolemy, the eternal the beloved of Phtah, a God illustrious a lord most excellent.

125.

called another name for him Ptolemy the deliverer of Egypt. the likeness of him who is Ptolemy - - -

Line 7th.

- all Egypt. shall serve those statues three times each day and place ornaments (or (drapery)) before them making offerings to them of adoration, appointed for their worship, as they do for the Gods of the country (on) the principal day of Panagyries, on the feast day, and on the day celebrated as his - which is the divine birthday, dedicating to the king of Egypt - Ptolemy - - -

Line 8th.

- statue of pure gold in all the chief houses of the land in Egypt, in the sanctuary, with shrines of the Gods of the country. So as for him on the day of grand Panagyries (ie.) of the going out of the God in the pure house of his statue; afterwards for them to carry in the appointed manner, raising them the shrine and statue of the God

91. [Hale, Jones, and Morton], *Report of the Committee . . . to Translate the Inscription on the Rosetta Stone.* Chromolithograph.

91. [Charles Reuben Hale, S. Huntington Jones, and Henry Morton]: *Report of the Committee Appointed by the Philomathean Society of the University of Pennsylvania to Translate the Inscription on the Rosetta Stone.* [Philadelphia: L. N. Rosenthal], 1858.

Chromolithograph

The first full translation of the Rosetta Stone, undertaken by three members of the University of Pennsylvania faculty, provided the basis for a notable display of chromolithographic book illustration by the Philadelphia lithographer, Louis Rosenthal. The entire book was lithographed, presumably to better accommodate the hieroglyphs, but Rosenthal went far beyond necessity. He created hundreds of crude but exuberant chromolithographs intermingled with the text, showing scenes from Egyptian life or elaborate borders in quasi-Egyptian motifs. It is one of the few American books printed entirely by lithography.

92. Oscar H. Harpel: *Harpel's Typograph or Book of Specimens Containing Useful Information, Suggestions and a Collection of Examples of Letterpress Job Printing Arranged for the Assistance of Master Printers, Amateurs, Apprentices, and Others.* Cincinnati: Oscar H. Harpel, 1870.

Electrotype and color printing from type and ornaments

Harpel's book provides a good survey of the state of the art in American letterpress printing in 1870. His handbook contains numerous examples of color printing both typographically and employing electrotypes, combined with instructions for their use in the press room. Harpel advises that the ability to print in multiple colors is "now generally expected of job printers."

93. Leon J. Fremaux: *New Orleans Characters.* [New Orleans]: Pychard & Garcia, 1876.

Hand-colored lithograph

Costume books and illustrations of typical trades and occupations, so common in European color plate books, are comparatively rare in America. This book of New Orleans street characters may be the best example of the genre printed in the United States. It is not surprising that it was produced in the most European of American cities.

94. Genevieve, Virginia, and Howard Jones: *Illustrations of the Nests and Eggs of Birds of Ohio....* Circleville, Ohio: [The Authors], 1879–1886.

Hand-colored lithograph

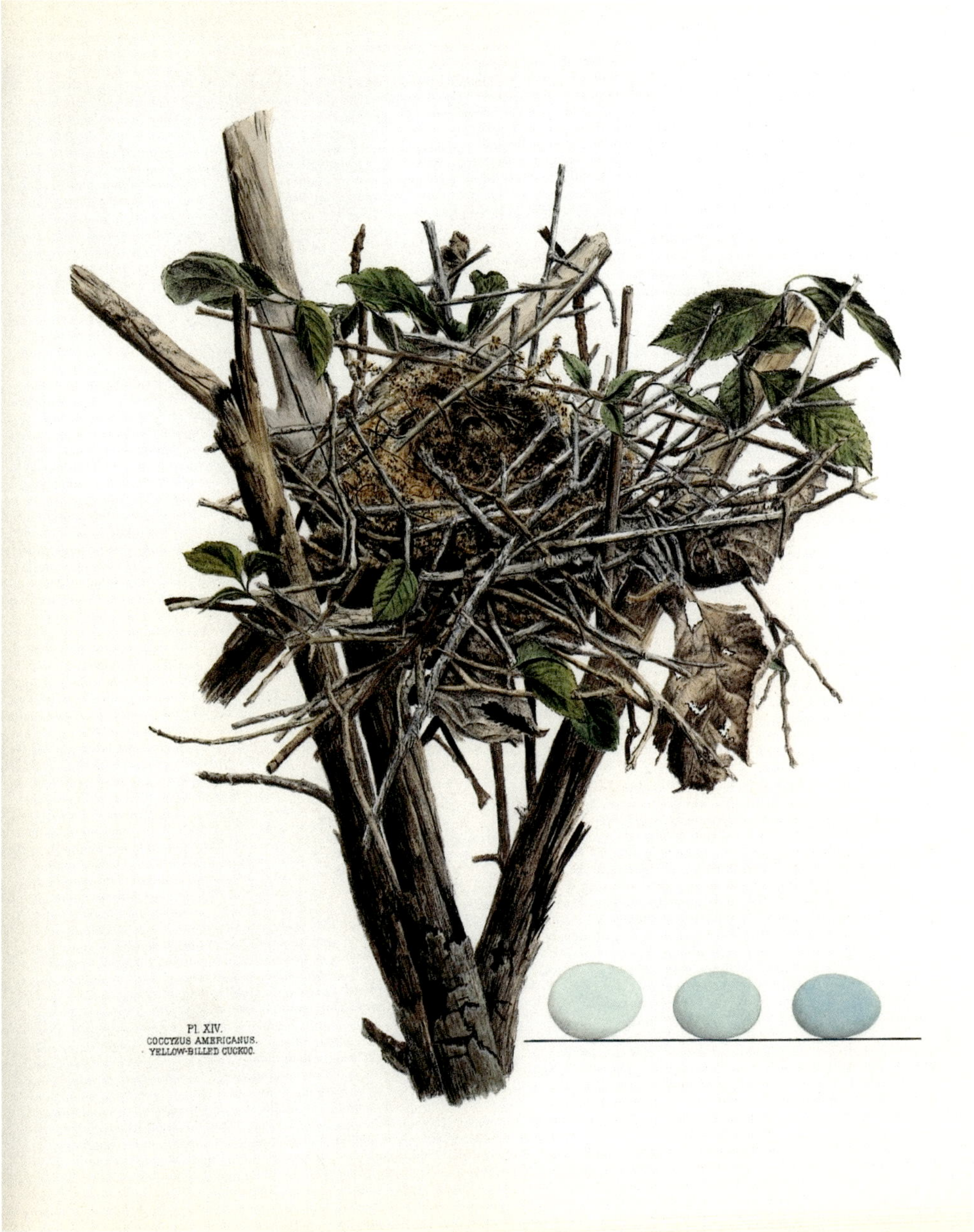

94. Genevieve and Jones, *Illustrations of the Nests and Eggs of Birds of Ohio....* Hand-colored lithograph.

This remarkable book was literally produced at home by members of the Jones family. The project was originally conceived by Genevieve Jones, a self-taught ornithologist and artist, who prepared the first lithographic stones in the living room of the Jones home in Circleville. The stones were then shipped to Cincinnati to be printed, and the plates returned for coloring. After Genevieve's untimely death from typhoid, her mother and brother completed the work over seven years with the help of several local colorists. No more than ninety sets were produced of this extraordinary labor of love, widely praised for its accuracy of depiction.

95. Alfred Tennyson: *The Lady of Shalott. Decorated by Howard Pyle.* New York: Dodd Mead & Company, 1881.

Chromotypograph

The Howard Pyle illustrations in this American edition of *The Lady of Shalott* were executed by the New York printer, Alphonse Brett, using metal relief blocks. Different surface treatments of the blocks could produce differing textures and patterns in the colors of the final product. This work was one of the most popular gift books of the late 19th century and was reissued many times. Similar methods were used in other artist-illustrated books at the end of the century.

96. Louis Prang: *Prang's Standard Alphabets.* Boston: Louis Prang, 1886.

Chromolithograph

The foremost practitioner of chromolithography in its heyday was Louis Prang of Boston. Prang was interested in every aspect of printing in color, and produced a number of handbooks such as this one, offering a menu of both engraved and lithographed alphabets with "regard for modern taste in lettering and decoration."

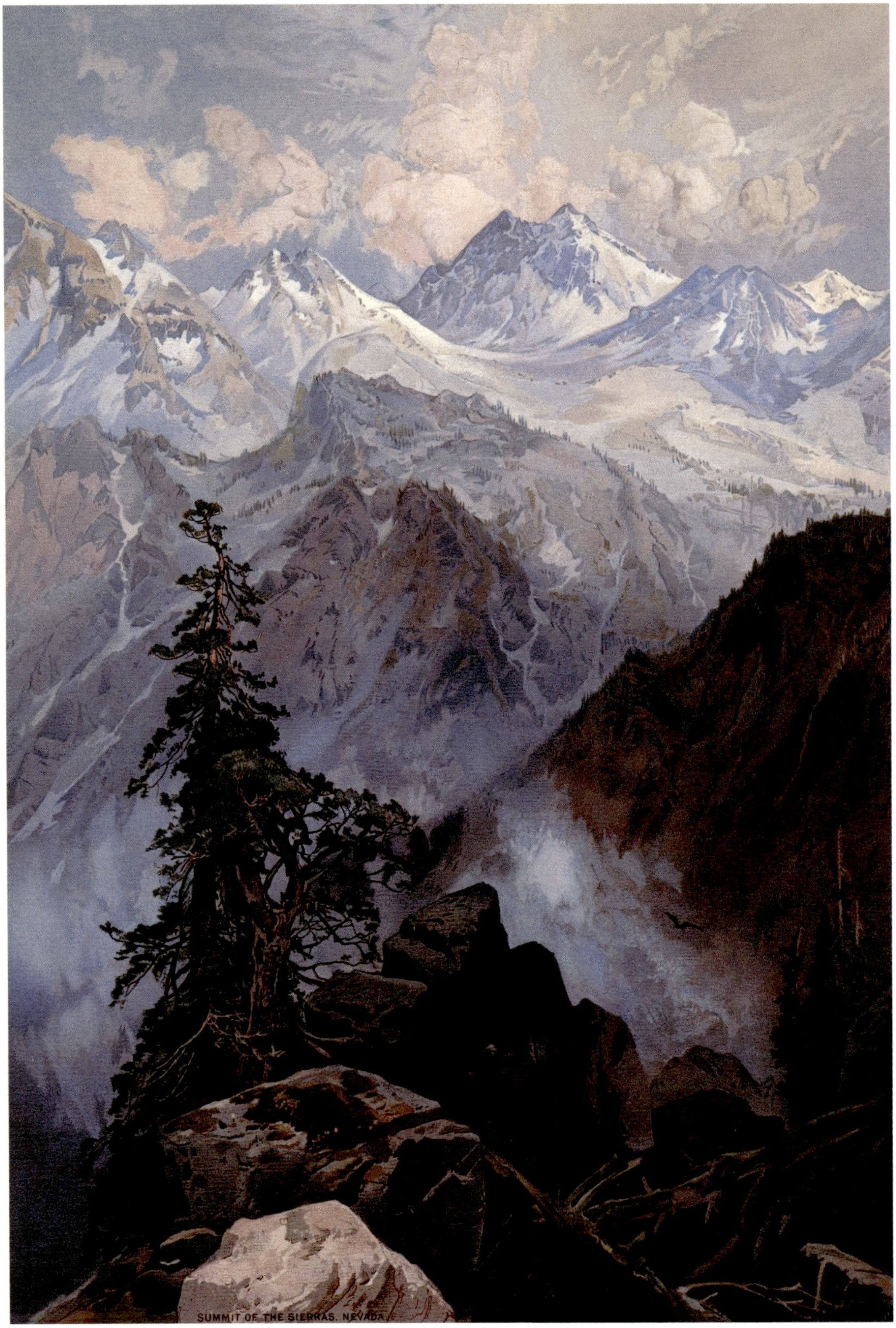

99. Hayden and Moran, *The Yellowstone National Park....*
Chromolithograph.

CASE 9: The Golden Age of Chromolithography 1862–1897

By the 1860s the advancing quality and lower cost of chromolithography had all but eliminated hand coloring in book illustration. As lithographers achieved increasingly subtle effects by overprinting colors with multiple stones, it became common to use a dozen or more in a complex print, each requiring a separate press run and mastery of exact registration. In the hands of a master such as Louis Prang, the results were sensational. A political refugee from Germany in 1848, Prang worked on fashion plates with Frank Leslie before starting his own Boston firm in 1858. He became a pioneer in every aspect of color printing, and his name is probably more often associated with the vast amounts of ephemera his firm produced than with book illustration. By the end of the century, however, he was indisputably the greatest printer and publisher of books with chromolithographic illustration, bringing the craft to its highest level of achievement.

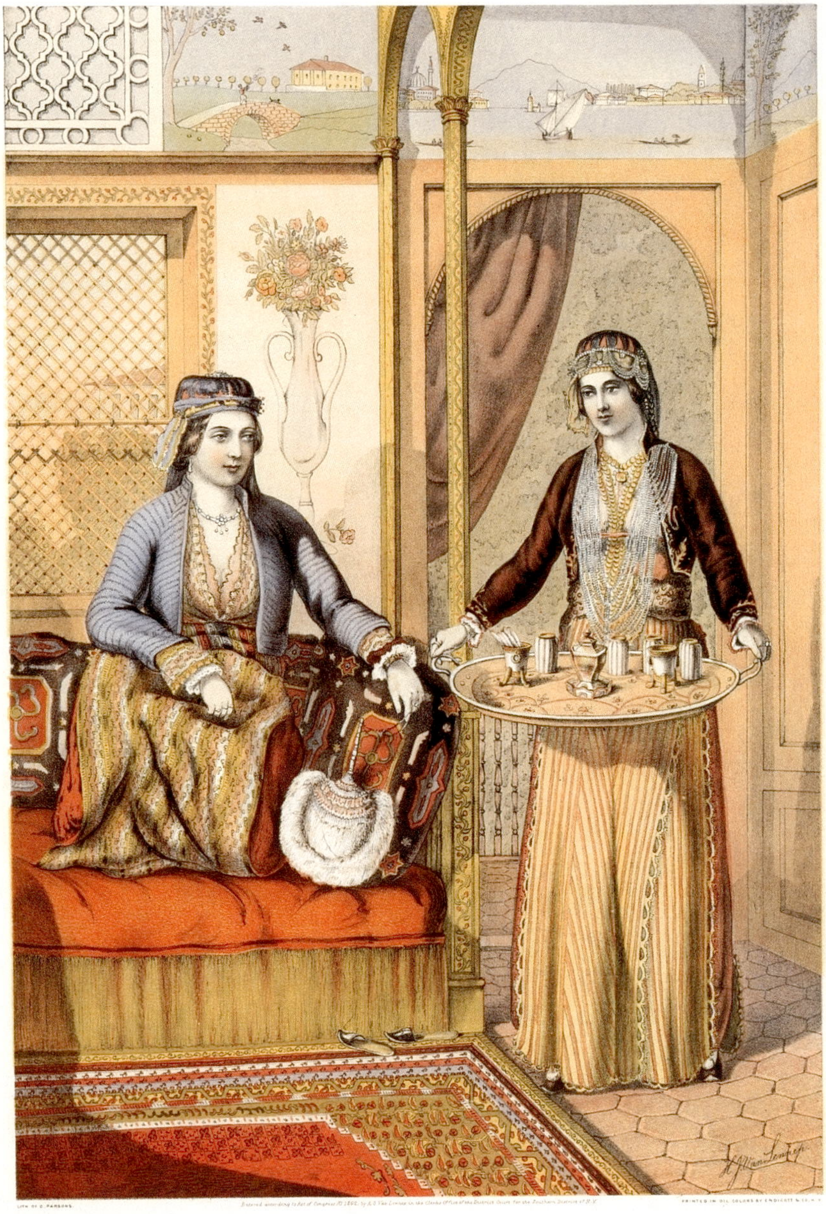

97. Van Lennup, *The Oriental Album.* Chromolithograph.

97. Henry J. Van Lennup: *The Oriental Album. Twenty Illustrations in Oil Colors of the People and Scenery of Turkey. . . .* New York: Anson D. F. Randolph, 1862.

Chromolithograph

This is one of the few large-scale chromolithographic works produced in the 1860s, a period when the Civil War seems to have curtailed the ambitions or markets of many printers. The New York lithographer, Endicott, achieved a rich variety of color which demonstrated the increased technical ability of American printers in the medium. The exotic views of harem life seem rather racy for mid-Victorian America.

98. [Colgate & Co.],
Illustrated Price List. . . .
Chromolithograph.

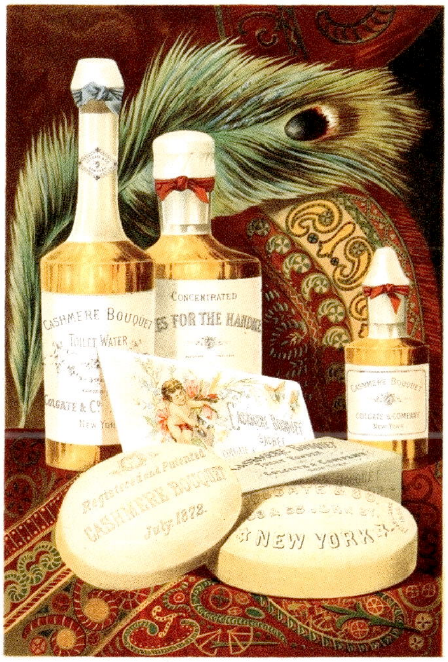

98. [Colgate & Company]: *Illustrated Price List of the Leading Styles of Toilet Soaps and Perfumery Manufactured by Colgate & Company.* New York: [Mayer, Merkel & Ottmann], [1872].

Chromolithograph

Some of the most elaborate chromolithographic works were trade catalogues. The high cost of producing such material, often in full-scale books, illustrates the degree to which consumer product makers were willing to spend on advertising even in the 19th century. This handsome Colgate catalogue contains thirty-four full-page chromolithographs in glowing color by the lithographers, Mayer, Merkel & Ottmann of New York, advertising various toiletry articles and soaps. Such catalogues were aimed mainly at the buyers for dry goods and department stores rather than the final consumer.

99. Ferdinand V. Hayden and Thomas Moran: *The Yellowstone National Park and the Mountain Regions of Portions of Idaho, Nevada, Colorado & Utah. Described by Prof. F. V. Hayden . . . Illustrated by Chromolithographic Reproductions of Watercolor Sketches, by Thomas Moran. . . .* Boston: L. Prang & Co., 1876.

Chromolithograph

This spectacular portfolio is one of the most famous of American color plate books, and the greatest American landscape book of the post-Civil War era. Although based on the work of an official government project, the Hayden Survey, it was issued as a commercial publication by Louis Prang. Thomas Moran's delicate treatments of the extraordinary colors of Yellowstone were successfully rendered into chromolithographs by Prang, whose reputation was made by the book. It marked the beginning of his dominance of the finest American chromolithographic work in the last quarter of the century.

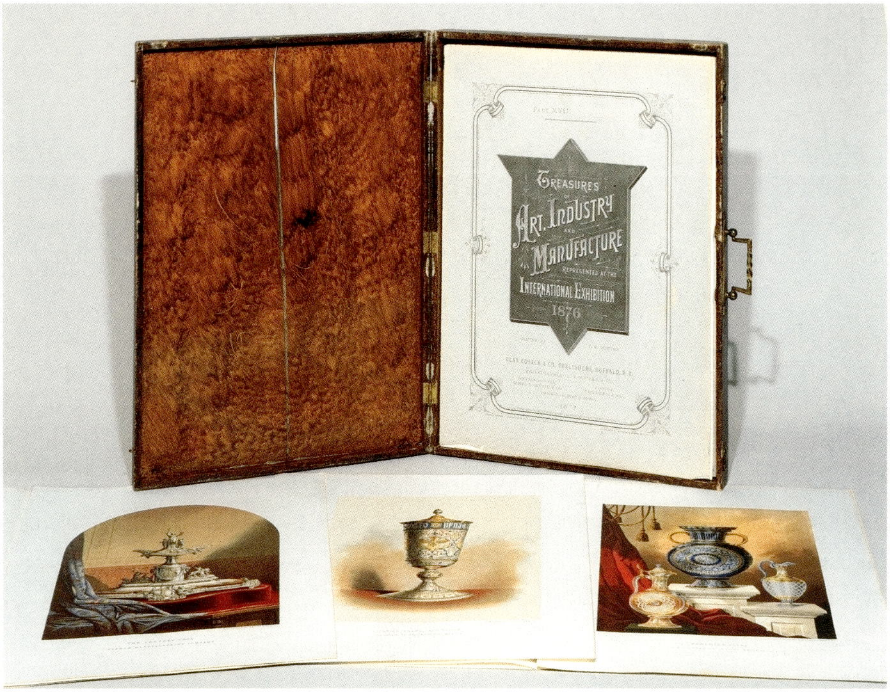

100. [Centennial Exposition], *Treasures of Art, Industry and Manufacture....*
Salesman's sample case.

100. [Centennial Exposition]: *Treasures of Art, Industry and Manufacture Represented at the International Exposition 1876.* Buffalo: Clay and Cosack, 1877–1878.

Chromolithograph

Produced by the firm of Clay, Cosack of Buffalo, this portfolio illustrates arts, crafts, and manufactures displayed at the Philadelphia Centennial Exposition of 1876. At its best, it represents some of the most delicate chromolithographic work done in America up to the time. A book such as this was far from cheap. The thirty-five parts cost two dollars each, or the equivalent of several thousand dollars in modern purchasing power. Such large color projects remained very expensive throughout the century, limiting their circulation to the most affluent segment of society.

101. [United States Navy]: *Regulations Governing the Uniform of the Commissioned Officers, Warrant Officers and Enlisted Men of the Navy of the United States.* Washington, D. C.: Government Printing Office, 1886.

Chromolithograph

Numerous military costume books appeared after the Civil War. Unlike the antebellum examples, almost all were published by the government. Richly illustrated manuals were issued by the Army and Navy to show proper military dress. This plate shows a variety of full dress and service uniforms for officers and other ratings.

102. F. Schuyler Mathews, ed.: *The Golden Flower Chrysanthemum.* Boston: Louis Prang, 1890.

Chromolithograph

Another Prang extravaganza, this book combines aspects of a gift book with snippets of poetry from various sources, a botanical work with plates of various species of chrysanthemums, and a wonderful example of American cloth binding. Many of the gift books of the end of the 19th century followed similar formats: small folios with poetry and chromolithographic plates alternating, in ornately stamped bindings. This is perhaps the most successful of the genre in its style and execution.

103. W. T. Walters and S. W. Bushell: *Oriental Ceramic Art. Collection of W. T. Walters. . . .* New York: D. Appleton & Co., 1897.

Chromolithograph

The catalogue of the great W. T. Walters collection of oriental porcelain, in ten large folios, contains 116 chromolithographs by Prang. It was his finest hour, and perhaps the greatest *tour de force* in chromolithography ever executed. Each plate required from twenty to forty-four stones to print, a staggering technical feat. The introduction to the set immodestly but accurately states that the plates "represent the highest type of work that has been produced in that branch of art." Even as his printed monument was being produced, Prang realized that new technologies were about to sweep the world of chromolithography away. In 1897 he merged his business with the Taber Art Company, specialists in photographic reproduction, and shortly thereafter retired.

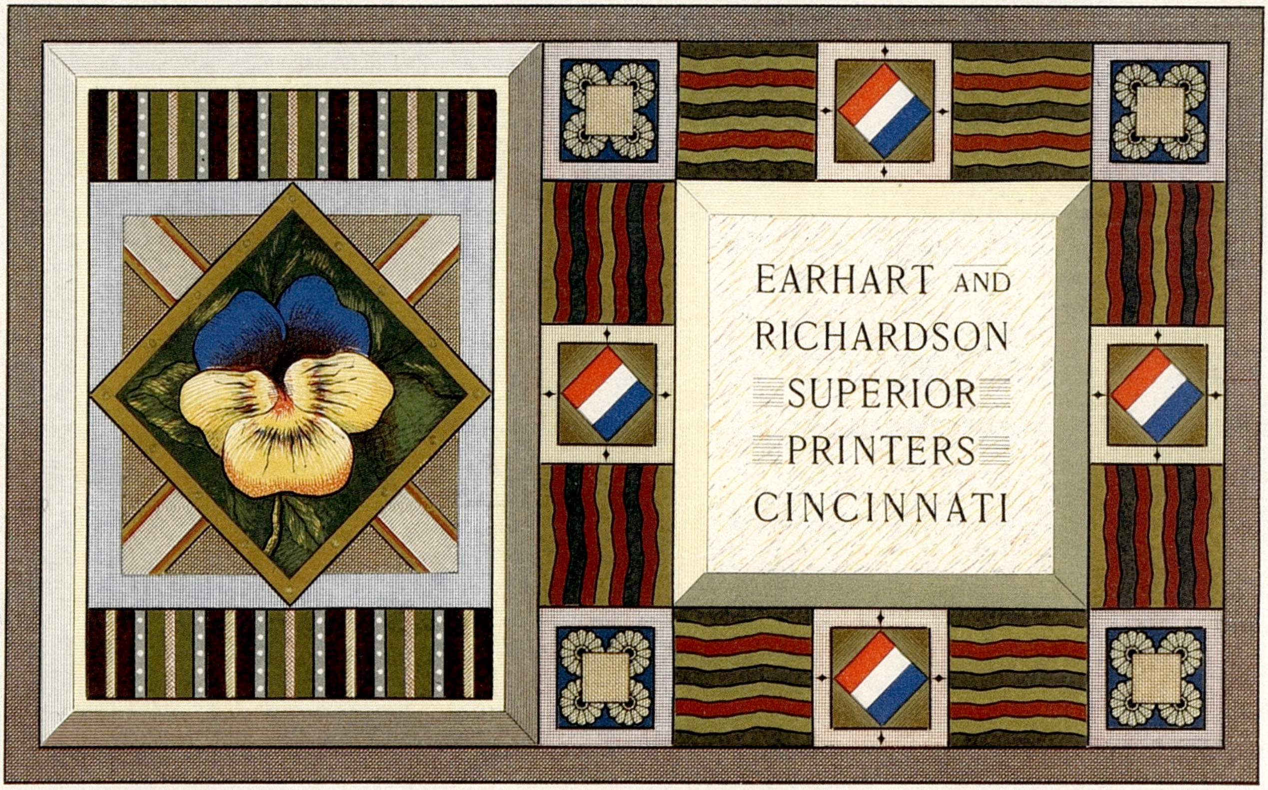

347

Card showing thirty-seven colors produced by six impressions. The colors were printed in the following order: Gold, Red, Blue, Yellow, Gray and Black. (See Plate 64).

111. Earhart, *The Color Printer*...
Chromotypograph.

CASE 10: The End of the Century 1884–1900

By the 1880s a broad range of processes were being used to create color book illustrations. The first part of this section juxtaposes four ways of approaching one topic, the illustration of butterflies. While one scientist, Edwards, clung to hand-colored lithographs as long as possible, and an amateur, Maynard, crudely produced his own plates in the same medium, another scientist, Scudder, embraced chromolithography. The fourth, Denton, managed to get excellent results from nature printing, but only by fanatical application.

Even as chromolithography reached its apogee in the 1890s, the technology which would replace it was developing rapidly. This was the trichromatic process which, by mixing and overprinting primary and secondary colors, could achieve a full spectrum of color with far fewer runs through the press than would be necessary in chromolithography. Combined with half-tone reproductions of photographs, the result was the beginning of the process which dominated color reproduction until the modern digital age. Although the final results were inferior to the best chromolithographic work in this early period, it was far cheaper. The successful coupling of the half-tone process with trichromatic color was the breakthrough. As the 19th century came to a close, it was clear that the days of chromolithography were numbered, and that the trichromatic half-tone (or four-color, as it became known with the addition of black) would rule the new century.

104. William H. Edwards: *The Butterflies of North America. Second Series.* Boston: Houghton, Mifflin and Company, 1884.

Hand-colored lithograph

Edwards' work was the last significant work of American natural history with plates made by hand coloring lithographs to the highest standards. Mrs. Lydia Bowen, a daughter of the Philadelphia lithographer, J. T. Bowen, and her sister, Mrs. Leslie, managed the production and hand coloring of the plates through the second volume of this work in 1884. When the third volume was issued in 1897, the plates were chromolithographs, and Edwards in his preface mourned the loss of "two such accomplished colorists as Mrs. Bowen and Mrs. Leslie, who had served their apprenticeship with Audubon – both of them now gone." The craft died with the last practitioners.

105. Charles J. Maynard: *The Butterflies of New England; with Original Descriptions of One Hundred and Six Species, Accompanied by an Appendix Containing Descriptions of One Hundred Additional Species....* Newtonville, Ma.: C. J. Maynard, 1891.

Hand-colored lithograph

By the last decade of the 19th century, the only remaining instances of hand-colored lithographs in books were stubborn individual practitioners such as Maynard, who gathered his own specimens, described them, drew his own stones, and oversaw their coloring. The result, although an interesting example of a determined eccentric, is a pale reflection of the old skills.

106. Samuel Scudder: *The Butterflies of the Eastern United States and Canada, with Special Reference to New England.* Cambridge: Printed for the author, 1889.

Chromolithograph

Unlike Edwards and Maynard, Scudder warmly embraced the new technologies of reproduction. His color plates of butterflies were produced by Thomas Sinclair of Philadelphia in chromolithography, using as many as fifteen stones to achieve color fidelity. Scudder's black and white plates used even more up-to-date technologies, such as gelatin process photographs, photogravures, and electrotypes. Sinclair also produced the chromolithographs for Edwards' final volume.

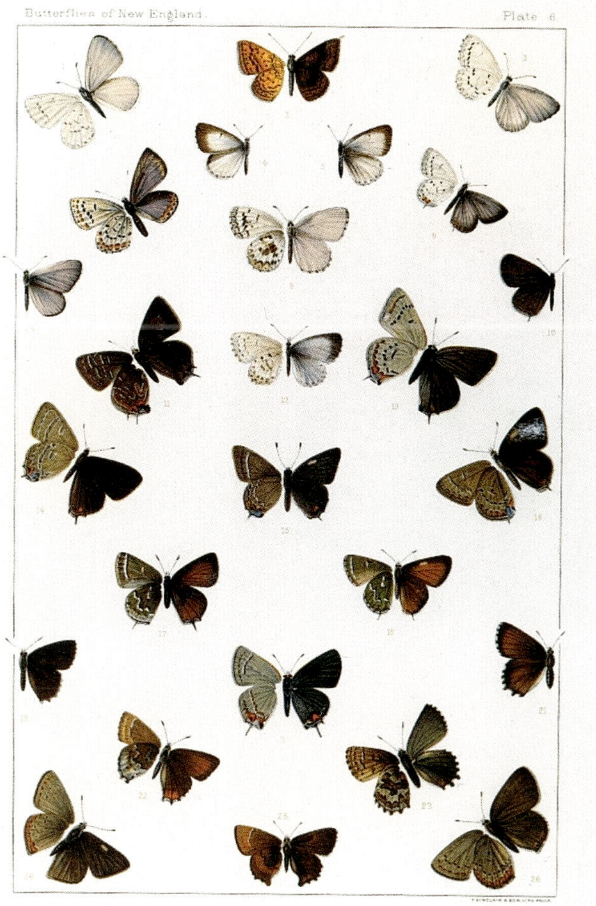

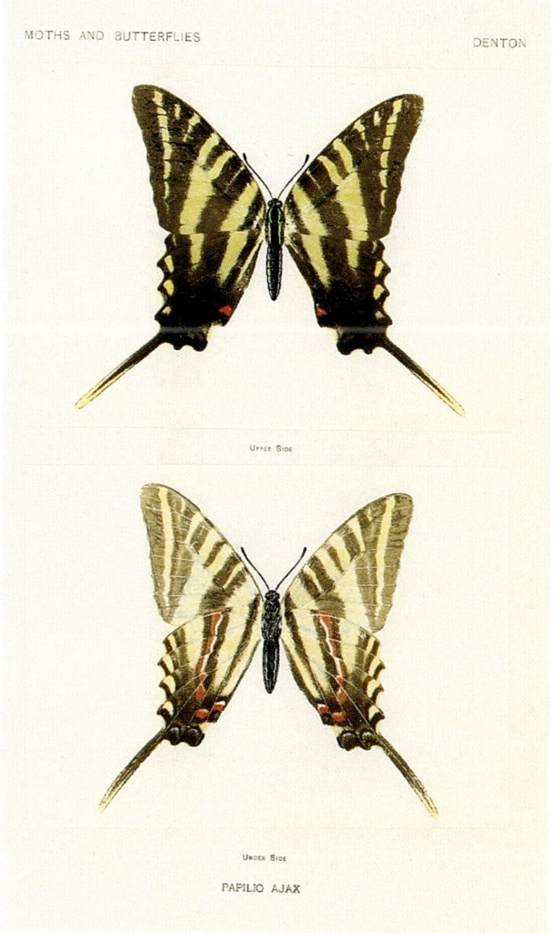

106. Scudder, *The Butterflies of the Eastern United States and Canada....* Chromolithograph.

107. Denton, *As Nature Shows Them....* Chromolithograph.

107. Sherman F. Denton: *As Nature Shows Them. Moths and Butterflies of the United States East of the Rocky Mountains.* Boston: Bradlee Whidden, 1900.

Transfer print from life, engraving with hand coloring

New methods of printing color, often too difficult to be practical, were sometimes undertaken by enthusiasts. Denton says the plates in this book "are direct transfers from the insects themselves; that is to say, the scales of the wings of the insects are transferred to the paper while the bodies are printed from engravings and afterward colored by hand...I have had to make over fifty thousand of these transfers for the entire edition, not being able to get anyone to help me who would do the work as I desired it done... I will say, however, that there never was a laborer more in love with his work...."

108. Celia Thaxter: *An Island Garden. With Pictures and Illuminations by Childe Hassam.* Cambridge: Riverside Press, 1894.

Chromolithograph

One of the most appealing books from the end of the century, this work celebrates the poet and patron of the arts, Celia Thaxter, and her garden on the Isle of Shoals on the Maine coast. The artist, Childe Hassam, a regular visitor and close friend of Thaxter, painted some of his most delightful pieces there. His illustrations in this book are among the few color illustrations in a 19th-century American book by an artist of renown who was not engaged in natural history or science. Armstrong & Company, the Boston firm responsible for the chromolithography, made a specialty of interpreting watercolors in chromolithography.

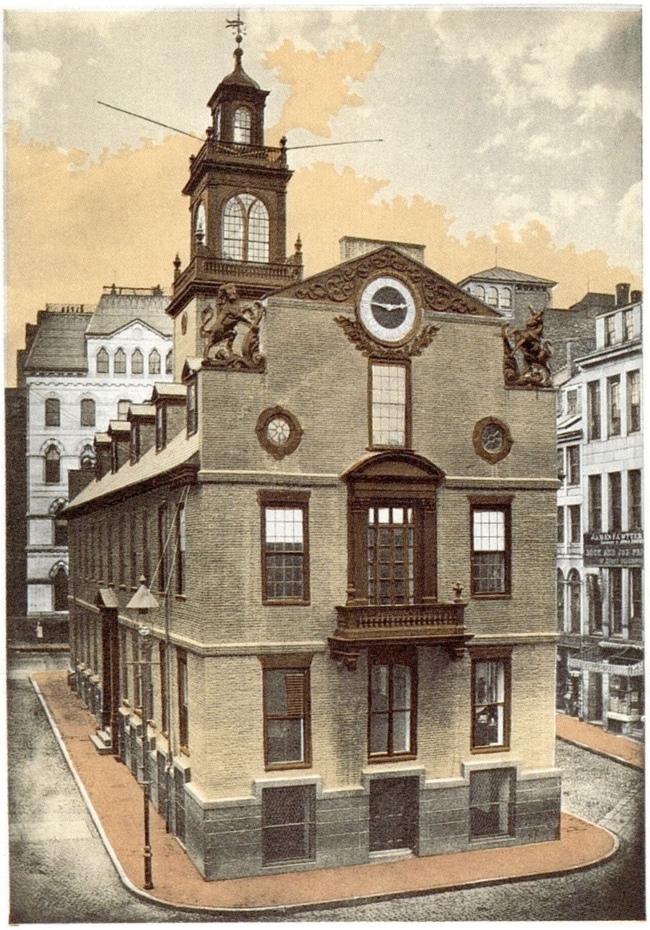

HELIO-CHROME HELIOTYPE PRINTING CO., BOSTON.

OLD STATE HOUSE

109. Whitefield, *The Homes of Our Forefathers....* Heliochrome.

109. Edwin Whitefield: *The Homes of Our Forefathers, in Boston, England.* [with:] *Homes of Our Forefathers in Boston, New England.* Boston: E. Whitefield, 1889.

Heliochrome

Various photographic mediums were increasingly used in color book illustration from the mid-1880s. Whitefield illustrated most of his books on colonial New England with chromolithographs, but in this publication he included a new process invented by the Heliotype Printing Company of Boston, printing color on top of a photographic image. The plate has an oddly three-dimensional quality.

110. Dr. Wilhelm Von Bezold: *The Theory of Color in its Relation to Art and Art-Industry.* Boston: L. Prang and Company, 1876.

Chromotypograph

Understanding the theory of primary colors and how they could be mixed to form other tones became increasingly important as chromolithography became more complex. It was essential for anyone attempting to master the three-color processes which came to the fore in the 1890s. Von Bezold was among the first scientists to offer a popular explanation of the pragmatic discoveries of Chevreul and the most recent scientific explorations. He sought to reach out to art and industry to explain color theory and its practical applications to society. Originally published in Germany in 1874, it should come as no surprise that Louis Prang published the first American edition.

111. John F. Earhart: *The Color Printer. A Treatise on the Use of Colors in Typographic Printing.* Cincinnati: Earhart and Richardson, 1892.

Chromotypograph

Earhart's treatise on color printing describes the evolving science of mixing and overprinting colors to obtain superb results from a variety of relief printing processes. Half-tone relief blocks were already being used, in combination with older wood and metal blocks, type, and typographic ornaments, to create a complex array of effects. The possibilities of the three-color process, which offered a far cheaper method of color printing than the multiple stones of chromolithography, were being systematized by printers such as Earhart on the eve of the half-tone revolution.

112. Arthur Mennell and Bruno Garlepp: *Bismarck Denkmal fur das Deutsche Volk.* Akron, Ohio: Werner Company, 1895.

Trichromatic half-tone

This massive memorial volume devoted to glorifying Otto von Bismarck contains some of the first trichromatic half-tone plates to appear in an American book. The Werner Company of Akron seems to have been at the forefront of new developments in printing technology at the end of the century. In this volume they reproduce with great technical skill, despite some obvious retouching to the original image, a very large photograph of the Iron Chancellor and the young Kaiser Wilhelm reviewing troops together. The combining of half-tone plates with the trichromatic color process offered a far cheaper way of producing color plates.

113. Dwight W. Huntington: *In Brush, Sedge, and Stubble. A Picture Book of the Shooting-Fields and Feathered Game of North America.* Cincinnati: The Sportsman's Society, 1898.

Trichromatic half-tone

Another pioneering use of colored half-tones as book illustration can be seen in this lavish picture book of hunting stories and pictures. In this instance the trichromatic half-tone process was used to reproduce paintings. They were printed by the Photo-Chromotype Engraving Company of Philadelphia. Within the next few years, the color half-tone process would move from the art folio and the lavish commemorative volume to become the primary means of color illustration.

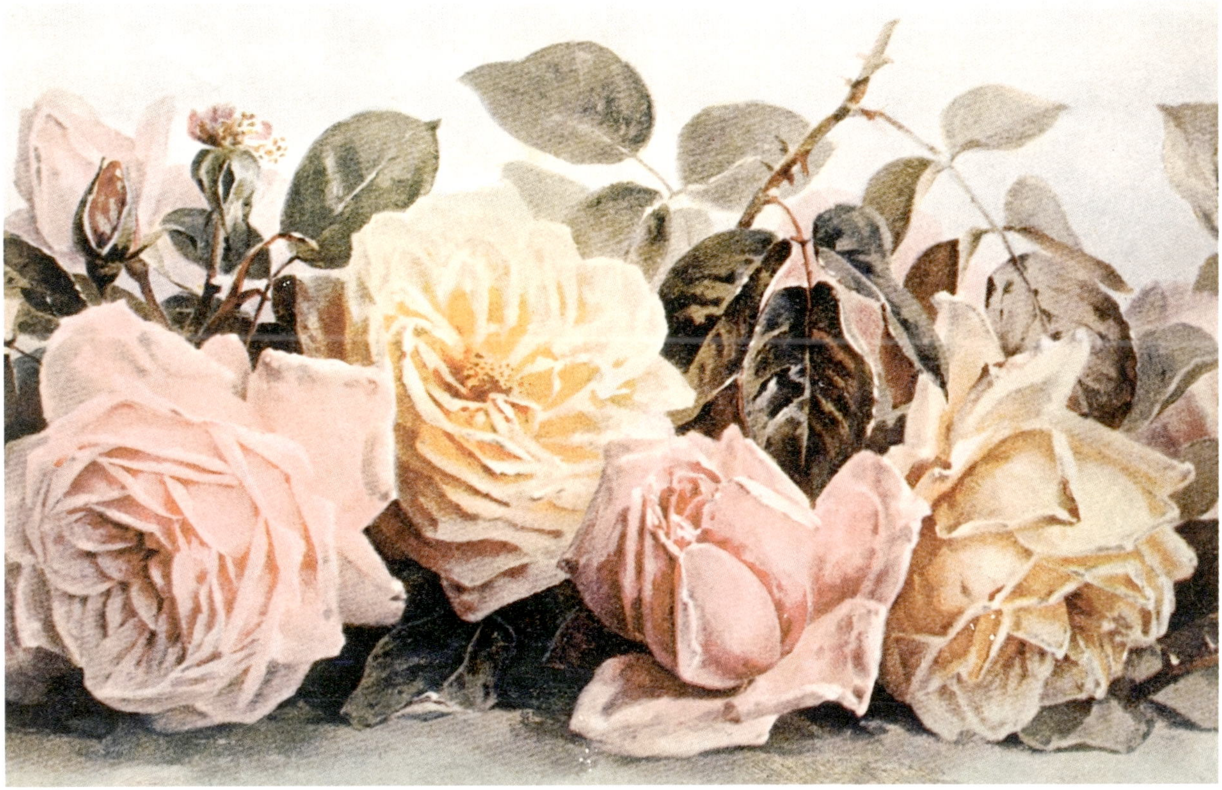

107. Sheldon,
The Practical Colorist....
Trichromatic half-tone.

114. Frederick M. Sheldon: *The Practical Colorist. A Pathfinder for the Artist Printer.* Burlington, Vt.: Owl Press, 1900.

Trichromatic half-tone

Sheldon attempted to instruct printers in the same basic principles of color which Earhart had discussed. Since the latter's book, however, the color half-tone process had fully come into its own, and much of this work is devoted to the new technology. "The newness, mystery, and uncertainty of the process keeps many printers from attempting three-color work," the author states, and indeed he finds that "one person's experience often apparently contradicts another's." But the advantages of being able to print all color from three plates by preparing the plates photographically would soon override all tentativeness. The 20th century would be ruled by the half-tone.

ACKNOWLEDGEMENTS

ANY EXHIBITION is really the work of many hands. A collector in a given field, or the curator of a show such as this, has innumerable debts to the many people who offered books or suggested themes, and to the friends who shared knowledge and enthusiasm. I have been fortunate in having generous friends and colleagues.

My greatest debt as a collector of American color plate books is to Michael Zinman, himself a great collector in many areas of American printing and book production. Having urged me to undertake a collection in the first place, he has assiduously acquired unusual items on my behalf with all of his extraordinary ability to find nuggets of gold in mounds of dross. Leonard Milberg, another superlative collector, encouraged me to pursue this project in its early stages. Jay Last, certainly the leading collector of early American color printing, has also been generous with his knowledge.

Among dealers, Charles Wood III has taken an interest in this project from the beginning, and has been most helpful in his advice on the details of the exhibition and catalogue. Donald Heald has loaned key items, and has shared his vast knowledge of original color. Clarence Wolf has found for me some of the most important items in my collection, and has constantly been on the lookout for more obscure pieces. I am deeply indebted to all of my colleagues in the antiquarian book trade who have found me books, offered me books, sold me books, and told me about books.

The Yale University Library has been invaluable as a reference source for this catalogue, and has also lent generously to the exhibition. I am particularly grateful to George Miles of the Beinecke Rare Book and Manuscript Library at Yale for his assistance. Georgia Barnhill at the American Antiquarian Society provided many useful suggestions for the catalogue. Ron Tyler of the Texas State Historical Society was also helpful. My thanks as well to all the librarians around the country and in Europe who replied to my census queries on several major books.

This catalogue would not have been accomplished without the help of my colleagues at the William Reese Company, particularly Leslie Warner. John Stinson and Joe Bray also provided assistance. Eric Holzenberg of The Grolier Club made several trips to New Haven to assist in the planning for the show. Both he and Carol Rothkopf were devoted proofreaders. Of course, any errors of fact or interpretation to be found here are entirely my own.

Finally, I thank my mother and late father, to whom this catalogue is dedicated. Many years ago they bought me my first rare book—an American color plate book–and set me on a happy course in the world of antiquarian books.

INDEX